Chair Yoga for Seniors Over 60

The Step-by-Step Guide with Cardio Exercises to Awaken Vitality Discover the Easiest 10-Minute Illustrated Routines and Strengthen Balance, Mobility and Flexibility

By

David Clem

The trademarks used are without any consent, and the trademark publication is without permission or backing by the trademark owner. All trademarks and brands within this book are for clarifying purposes only, owned by themselves, and not affiliated with this document.

Contents

Introduction

Thank you for visiting "Chair Yoga for Wellness and Wellbeing." This book is your thorough guide to chair Yoga and its advantages. This book will provide the information and resources you need to improve your physical and emotional well-being through chair yoga, whether you're completely new to Yoga or a seasoned practitioner.

A modified version of conventional Yoga known as "chair yoga" enables people to practice Yoga while sitting or with the assistance of a chair. It provides a mild and approachable method for improving posture, flexibility, and strength, lowering stress levels, and encouraging relaxation. Chair yoga is unique because it is accessible to individuals of various ages, abilities, and fitness levels. Seniors, office workers, those with restricted mobility, and others looking to develop a mindful practice may all benefit greatly.

We explore the fundamental ideas and methods of chair yoga in this book, giving readers a thorough comprehension of its underpinnings. You will learn how Yoga in chairs differs from conventional Yoga and its origins, and how it has changed and evolved through time. You will better understand the core of chair yoga and its distinctive method of well-being.

Chair yoga has advantages that go beyond good physical wellness. You may have better mental and emotional health through frequent practice, including less stress, sharper attention, and a sensation of relaxation. Additionally, we examine the benefits of chair yoga for various demographics, including the elderly, office workers, and those with restricted mobility, emphasizing how it can be customized to match their unique requirements and improve their general level of life.

This book makes chair yoga accessible for beginners. We advise setting up a good practice area, choosing the appropriate chair and devices, and ensuring safety by adjusting and using the necessary breathing methods. The idea is to give you the confidence and comfort to practice chair yoga.

Throughout this book, you'll find thorough directions and images for various postures and exercises, making you comfortable with the right alignment and form. We also provide a recommended training program to walk you through incorporating chair yoga into your regular practice. This program contains a daily routine that lasts 10 minutes and may be altered to fit your needs and tastes.

The book "Chair Yoga for Wellness and Wellbeing" aims to be a useful and educational resource. Its design is a learning tool and a clear road map for the chair's yoga experience. This book provides helpful ideas, strategies, and motivation to help you reach your objectives, including improving physical fitness, managing stress, or developing a stronger mind-body connection.

So come along as we investigate the healing effects of chair yoga. Accept the advantages it gives, and you'll find a way to better health and a more peaceful existence. Prepare to settle into a comfortable position, connect with your respiration, and begin a rewarding chair yoga practice.

Section 1: Introduction and Benefits of Chair Yoga

Chapter 1: Yoga Chair

The mild practice known as "chair yoga" consists of asanas (postures) carried out while seated and with a chair. Chair yoga sessions are typically designed for people who have physical limitations or are above 50 and find a traditional yoga session too difficult. It is also an excellent style of Yoga for newbies or those who want to concentrate on a milder practice. It is even possible to add aspects of Chair yoga into a typical Hatha yoga practice, particularly to assist people who struggle with balance or anyone who has difficulty going down on the floor and back up again.

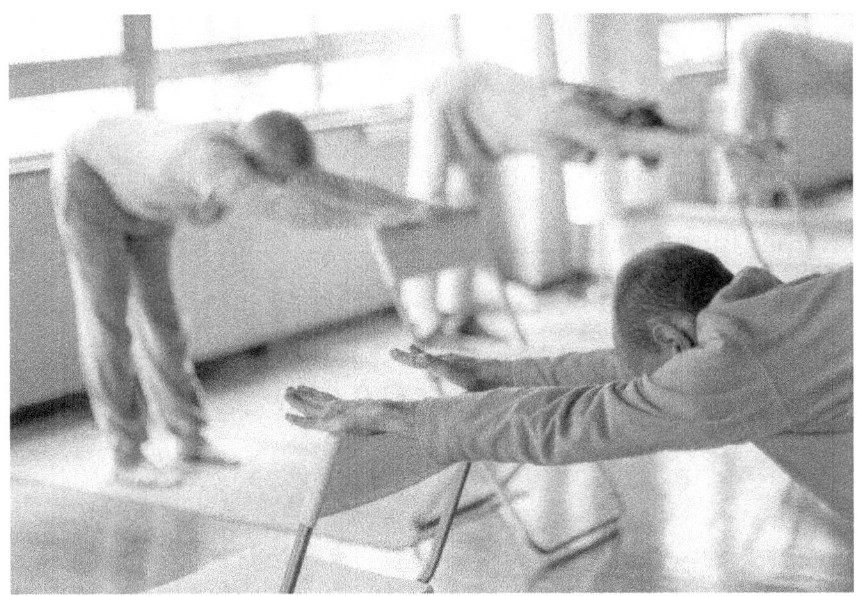

The benefits of flexibility, strength, and increased body awareness from regular yoga practice are also derived from chair yoga. In Chair Yoga classes, standing poses are sometimes incorporated, and a seat is used to assist with and enhance balance during these standing postures. In addition to pranayama breathing methods and meditation, Yoga in a chair may also involve these practices to help participants relax, concentrate, and gain mental clarity. Backbends, twists, hip openers, and forward folds are traditional yoga poses that can be adapted to practice while seated in a chair. For instance, in the seated variation of the mountain position, the yogi will have their feet planted firmly on the ground while their knees will be bent at a ninety-degree angle. Afterward, the palms of the hands are turned toward the sky as the arms are elevated overhead. The eyes meet in the middle of the palms.

Another fundamental yoga position, the forward fold, can be executed either while seated on a chair or standing, with the hands gripping the rear portion of the backrest for support. Yoga has several well-documented advantages, including reducing pain and improving flexibility. As a result, more than 90 percent of Americans exercise Yoga for their health and wellness should not come as a surprise. Traditional Yoga may be challenging for certain people, particularly those with limited mobility or who suffer from chronic diseases such as arthritis or heart disease. Yoga practice, while seated, can, thankfully, serve as an alternative. It is a form of Yoga that uses seated positions to make it more approachable. Continue reading to find out more regarding chair yoga, including important places that you can do to get started.

1.1: History

Chair yoga was developed in 1982 by yoga instructor Laxmi Voelker-Binder to make traditional Yoga more accessible to students with arthritis. Traditional yoga poses (known as asanas), mental concentration (known as dyana), and breathing exercises (known as pranayama) are all included in chair yoga.

On the other hand, standard yoga poses are altered in gentle practice so that they can be performed while seated in a chair. Alternatively, you might use a seat to help you maintain your balance while executing standing positions. The vast majority of yoga positions, including twists, backbends, and back folds, are amenable to modification for chair yoga. You can take a chair yoga class or a more traditional form incorporating sitting adjustments according to your capabilities.

1.2: Advantages

Traditional yoga postures use the same muscles as their modified chair yoga counterparts. Therefore, inclusive practice offers comparable positive effects on health. One benefit of chair yoga is that it can help balance and flexibility. One's health and well-being need to keep their equilibrium and maintain their flexibility. It can both lessen the likelihood of you being injured and make it easier to maintain your independence as you age. This is extremely important because three million older persons visit the emergency room yearly with injuries sustained from falls. In a study conducted in 2010, seniors living in a retirement facility practiced Yoga biweekly for one year. The majority of the poses were accomplished either while they were seated in an ottoman or while they were standing supported by a chair for stability. The subjects improved their lower-body flexibility and static balance when the experiment was over. They also experienced a decreased fear of slipping and had more trust in their ability to move about physically. Individuals of all ages may experience gains in their strength after practicing traditional Yoga. And under a review published in 2021, chair yoga can assist older persons in building and preserving their muscle power. Researchers have discovered exercises performed while seated benefit the upper and lower body. This is significant because, as people become older, their muscular mass naturally decreases. This deterioration may also be associated with losing power and mobility in people in their later years.

There is some evidence that regular yoga practice can give an advantage to upgrades in mental health, such as lower levels of anxiety and a more positive disposition. Evidence shows that these advantages apply to various yoga practices, including chair yoga. Participants in a pilot trial on a smaller scale were asked to attend chair yoga lessons once per week. After three months, participants reported changes such as lower stress levels, improved mood, and a reduction in the number of panic attacks they had. In addition, they improved their general health, physical wellness, and emotional and social well-being.

People with chronic health concerns like diabetes of the type 2 variety may find that seated Yoga helps them manage their condition. For instance, a brief pilot study investigated how persons with diabetes responded to participating in a chair yoga session that lasted for ten minutes. Participants got conventional medical treatment and were urged to make the habit a regular part of their lives. Following up with them after three months, we found that their blood sugar levels, heart rates, and blood pressure had all improved. Roughly twenty percent of adults suffer from chronic pain, which can significantly impact how they go about their everyday lives. In addition, mounting evidence suggests Yoga could be a useful alternative treatment for managing chronic pain. One piece of research indicates that senior citizens who practice chair Yoga may experience less pain and exhaustion due to osteoarthritis.

1.3: Who Should Perform Chair Yoga?

Anyone may enjoy chair yoga. However, the revised procedure might be the best option for the following categories of people:

- People 66 and older: Chair yoga is a low-impact exercise suitable for older individuals and can help promote healthy aging. It may be especially intriguing to older persons due to its adaptability and benefits, including a lower risk of falling and improved mobility in practical situations.

- People who live with persistent medical conditions: A growing body of evidence suggests that practicing seated Yoga might assist people in managing chronic diseases (and the discomfort that is associated with them), including diabetes, osteoarthritis, and dementia.

- Individuals struggle with mobility because seated yoga postures allow them to reap the advantages of traditional Yoga even when they cannot stand for extended periods. For instance, it has been demonstrated that patients healing from spinal cord damage and those suffering from multiple sclerosis can benefit from chair yoga.

- Employees who spend their days at an office: An exhausted state, elevated blood pressure, and soreness in the back region, neck, and shoulders can be brought on by sitting behind a desk for an extended amount of time. There is some evidence that Yoga at work can help reduce back pain symptoms and improve mental health. According to the findings of one study, reducing stress in both the body and the mind with only fifteen minutes of practicing chair yoga at work is possible.

However, before beginning chair yoga, discussing the practice with your primary care physician is best, particularly if you suffer from medical conditions or concerns.

1.4: How Frequently Should You Participate in Chair Yoga Sessions?

No set recommendation can be found regarding how frequently one should engage in chair yoga. However, according to the CDC, persons 65 and older should participate in strengthening exercises twice weekly and balance activities thrice weekly. Therefore, incorporating two or three chair yoga sessions into your weekly routine could be a wonderful place to start.

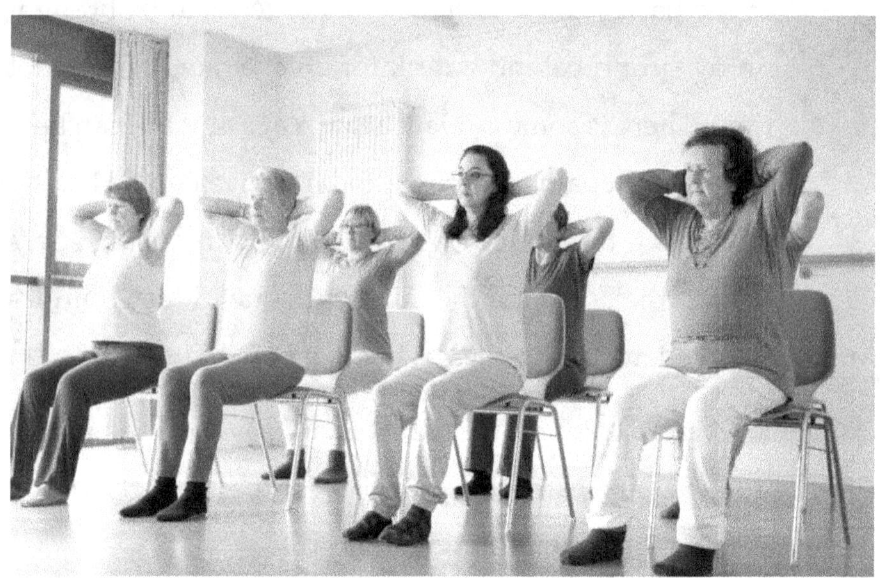

But remember that even a little physical activity is more advantageous than none. Studies have shown that even sporadic yoga practice can benefit elderly persons.

1.5: The Distinctive Characteristics of Chair Yoga in Contrast To Traditional Yoga

A renowned practice that dates back thousands of years, Yoga has been known for an exceptionally long time. It is a practice that aims to improve one's health on all fronts, including the physical, the mental, and the spiritual. Assorted styles of Yoga have developed over time to meet a comprehensive range of conditions and accommodate a variety of levels of physical ability. Yoga in a chair and traditional Yoga are well-known varieties of practice, yet they are quite different.

1. Accessibility

Accessibility is one of the utmost considerable factors differentiating Chair Yoga from Traditional Yoga. Using an exercise mat or a yoga mat designed specifically for the purpose, practitioners will move through a series of postures known as asanas. It calls for a certain degree of movement, balance, and flexibility on the part of the individual. On the other side, Chair Yoga was developed especially for people with restricted mobility, physical limitations, or difficulty conducting Yoga on the floor. This type of Yoga has been increasingly popular in recent years. Chair Yoga involves doing various yoga postures and exercises while seated on a chair or with the assistance of a chair. Traditional yoga positions typically include the practitioner's body coming into physical contact with the ground or a yoga mat, which offers the body both support and stability. To maintain the postures and move fluidly through the sequences, practitioners rely on the stamina of their bodies.

On the other hand, Chair Yoga makes use of the support that the chair provides. Individuals who are physically restricted or have limited mobility can engage in Yoga without risk, thanks to the chair's capacity to provide stability, balance, or a sense of security. They can achieve modified poses by making the chair a component of their body, which provides a stable basis from which to work. The breadth of motion involved in traditional Yoga is significantly less engaged in chair yoga, another notable distinction between the two forms of Yoga. Traditional Yoga typically involves various moves that test one's flexibility, strength, and ability to maintain balance. Yogis will go from positions done standing to poses done sitting and even inverted at times. Traditional yoga movements are adapted for those with restricted mobility and practice Chair Yoga instead. It is possible that a person's range of motion will be determined, and the poses will be modified to be executed while seated in a chair. The practitioners of chair yoga can reap the advantages of Yoga without placing an undue amount of effort on their bodies.

2. Techniques of Breathing

The techniques of breathing, also known as pranayama, are an essential component of Yoga. Deep, diaphragmatic breathing, as well as particular techniques for breath control, are emphasized in traditional Yoga to recover the flow of energy during the body. In Chair Yoga, traditional breathing exercises are modified so that they may be performed while seated. Practitioners learn to center their attention on their breath and adopt various modified breathing routines that may be performed in a relaxed manner while sitting on a chair. Individuals who have difficulty moving around will still benefit from pranayama's relaxing and refreshing effects o.

Traditional yoga practices frequently center their attention on the relationship between the mind and the body as well as the process of spiritual development. They use meditation, praying, and mindfulness techniques to help people relax and become more aware of themselves. Although it retains certain aspects of traditional Yoga, Chair Yoga typically emphasizes overall physical health and movement that serves a purpose. Because it seeks to increase a person's strength, flexibility,

harmony, and general mobility, it is popular among senior citizens, people who have sustained injuries, and those seeking rehabilitation.

Yoga in chairs and traditional Yoga are quite different from one another in some important respects, including accessibility, assistance with physical activity, and range of action, breathing methods, and the primary intention of the practice. Yoga is made available to more people since it may be adapted into postures and exercises that can be carried out while seated in a chair. This broadens the audience that can participate in Yoga. On the other hand, traditional Yoga incorporates a much wider variety of postures, motions, and spiritual practices than modern Yoga. Hatha and Vinyasa yoga styles offer various health advantages, each of which can be tailored to the practitioner's specific requirements and capabilities.

Chapter 2: Benefits of Chair Yoga

Traditional Yoga, an age-old discipline with positions that go back more than 5,000 years, is where chair yoga originates. Most conventional yoga postures, if not all, may be performed while seated or stretching in a chair. Because of this, chair yoga is appropriate for people of all experience levels, even elders, and it's fun.

2.1: The Health Advantages of Chair Yoga

In addition to its many advantages, chair yoga is an excellent choice for less mobile users since it provides extra support while encouraging an active lifestyle. Chair yoga enhances your quality of life and balance, cooperation, and core strength, which is crucial for seniors more susceptible to losing equilibrium. Below are a few of the main advantages.

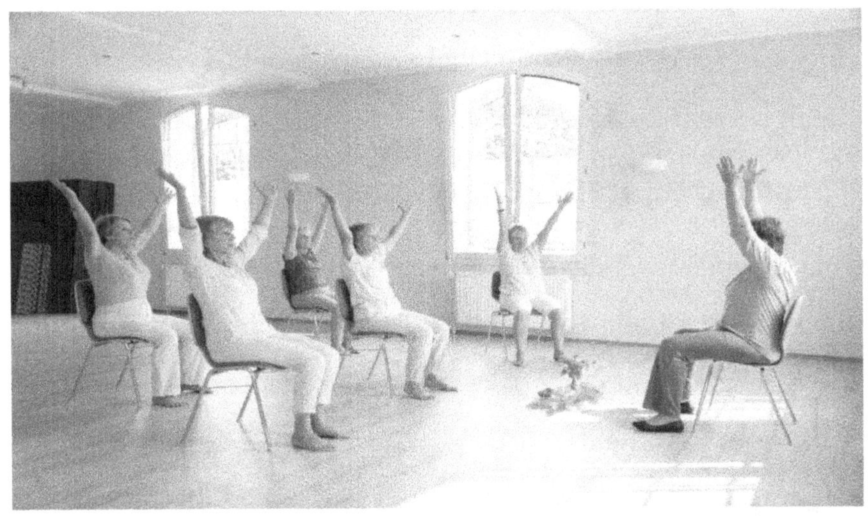

1: Enhanced Versatility

Improved flexibility is one of chair yoga's key advantages. Sitting on a chair allows you to concentrate on every motion and stretch, allowing you to maintain each posture for longer and get more profound freedom. Seniors at a greater risk of falling should focus on improving their range of motion by holding the poses for extended periods.

2: Better coordination and balance

The ability to develop balance and coordination is yet another important advantage of chair yoga. Keeping your equilibrium might become harder as you get older. Maintaining your freedom and participating in what you might be easier by developing balance and coordination.

To enhance your balance, practice chair yoga, where you may pay close attention to each motion and hold the postures for longer as necessary. Posing helps you develop core strength, which is great for older citizens.

3: Improved Heart Health

Chair yoga may help you enhance cardiovascular health by pushing your body to its limits. By increasing your flexibility and strength, you can strike the required positions with less effort from your heart.

4: Increasing power

Strengthening is also another significant advantage of chair yoga. Seniors who reside alone and wish to keep up with domestic duties should focus on building their strength. It's also a terrific approach for those who are handicapped or have limited mobility to gain independence daily.

5: Stress management

In addition to its physical advantages, chair yoga may help you de-stress. An excellent approach to center yourself and enhance your mental health is Yoga. Lowering your anxiety and stress may help you feel better about yourself, your mood, and your general view of life. Although they are sometimes disregarded, these advantages are among the main causes of why so many individuals like Yoga.

6: Capacity to Manage Pain

Chronic discomfort is among the hardest aspects of aging older. Chronic pain remains conceivable, even if you are physically fit, have decent flexibility, and follow a balanced diet.

Through an increase in endorphin release, chair yoga may aid in pain management. Your body's painkillers are endorphins, and chair yoga may help you lessen pain from chronic diseases or accidents.

Strengthening and increasing flexibility may also help lessen chronic pain. These advantages may assist you in avoiding the use of addictive painkillers and in finding more integrative solutions to your health problems.

7: Better Sleeping Conditions

For people who have trouble falling asleep, Yoga in a chair is a wonderful technique to enhance the quality of their sleep. Regular chair yoga sessions will help you naturally decrease the times you get up all night, making it simpler to stick to a daily schedule.

8: Reduce your vulnerability to chronic diseases

As many of these problems are linked to being overweight, exercise may help you prevent developing certain chronic disorders, including type 2 diabetes, bone loss, heart disease, several forms of cancer, anxiety and depression, and dementia. These long-term conditions may drastically reduce your standard of living and make it harder for you to receive the activity you need to be healthy.

9: Improved Alignment and Posture

The muscles that support your upright posture when sitting and standing may be strengthened with chair workouts. Good alignment and posture support your muscles, joints, bones, ligaments, and tendons while enhancing blood flow and maintaining the health of your blood vessels and nerves. You may maximize your potential for weight reduction by exercising with proper alignment and posture.

10: Helps to Improve Memory

Recent studies have shown that exercise boosts blood flow to two regions of the brain linked to memory, suggesting that chair exercises may help persons with Alzheimer's disease as well as other memory problems. Additionally, repetitious chair workouts force your brain to adopt a new habit, which improves memory. You may overcome midday slumps and mental exhaustion by exercising in a chair.

11: Boost your self-esteem and confidence.

Elderly people can have confidence issues, particularly after a major fall or after putting on weight. Exercise may help you feel more confident.

2.2: Chair Yoga's Benefits for Seniors

Chair yoga provides a variety of variants that are ideal even for individuals with restricted mobility because of its secure and gentle approach. For older men, Yoga offers a risk-free way to enjoy many advantages of an active lifestyle.

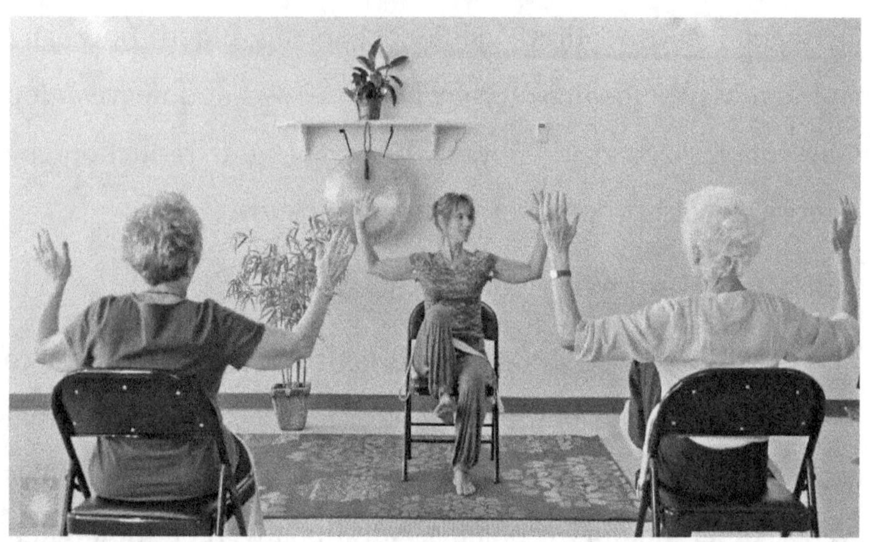

These consist of:

- Greater flexibility: The majority of everyday jobs need some degree of flexibility. Consequently, stretching, bending, and twisting each day is crucial. Chair yoga practitioners enhance mobility by pushing their bodies to keep and build flexibility.

- Muscular strength: Chair yoga may gradually increase muscular strength with each practice. This enhances balance and agility while protecting your body from harm.

- Improved proprioception, balance, and coordination: Proprioception is how your body moves in space. Your proprioception increases as you go from one posture to the next in a chair meditation sequence, improving your balance and coordination.

- Yoga naturally makes you aware of your respiration and movement, which helps divert your attention from stressful thoughts. The motions are soothing and even peaceful.

- Less pain and improved pain management techniques: Exercise in any form encourages the release of endorphins, our bodies' natural painkillers. Yoga and other forms of exercise have been demonstrated to drastically lower the number of painkillers consumed by patients with persistent backache. Additionally, the practice allows you to concentrate on your breathing and aids with pain management.

- Better sleep: Regular exercise, such as yoga chair poses, may boost your body's circadian rhythm and enhance the quality of your sleep. When the emphasis was placed on the quantity of sleep instead of the amount, around 55% of those who practice Yoga reported better sleep. The correct level of effort is provided by chair yoga without going beyond what is comfortable or comfortable. Ending the day with a restful night's sleep is made possible by doing this.

- Increases self-assurance and lessens melancholy and anxiety: Numerous studies have shown that Yoga helps alleviate the signs and symptoms of depression in persons of all ages, even those over 65.

2.3: The Advantages of Desk-Chair Yoga

What motivates you to practice chair yoga, then? The advantages of chair yoga for the body and mind are many. Here are some of chair yoga's main benefits:

1: Excellent for Those Who Find Traditional Yoga Difficult to Practice

Chair yoga is a terrific option for individuals who have trouble with regular Yoga, which is one of its key advantages. As we previously discussed, an arthritic yogi was the initial inspiration for the development of chair yoga.

This kind of Yoga is beneficial for those without arthritis as well. Further, it may help older people who find it difficult to do the up-and-down movements of conventional Yoga.

2: Perfect for Long Flights or Desk Jobs

If you haven't already heard, sitting has replaced smoking.

But what can you truly accomplish if you have a desk job?

According to University of Pennsylvania research, chair yoga helps ease the strain and stress of working at a desk all day.

You may benefit from mindful movement on long-haul flights and using it in the workplace. Due to the prolonged immobility seen on long-haul flights, blood clots are a possibility. You may increase blood flow and lower your risk of developing clots by Yoga while seated.

3: Each office is furnished with chairs. Save room!

You might not have enough room to set up a mat if you attempt to practice Yoga in a tiny place. It may be useful because chair yoga only requires a little space to practice.

Chair yoga practitioners may also continue to wear their regular office attire, saving time on getting dressed and, perhaps most crucially, preventing the sight of their manager in Lulu lemons.

Furthermore, seats are quite accessible. Most attendees have chairs they may use, while some businesses utilize the boardrooms or auditoriums on-site.

Not in the workplace? Chair yoga may be practiced on a plane, a park bench, a low brick wall, or while watching TV at home.

4: Enhanced Versatility

This is an excellent choice if you want to expand your flexibility. Flexibility is crucial for daily activities like tying your footwear together, picking up objects off the floor, and reaching high in your cabinets, even if you are not an athlete.

Biweekly yoga sessions have been shown to enhance balance and increase flexibility in research that lasted 10 weeks.

5: Increased Power

Most of us consider heavy lifting when we want to increase our strength. However, not everyone can engage in heavy lifting due to injuries or persistent discomfort.

6: Lessen Pain and Stress

Another excellent exercise for anyone wanting to relieve tension and discomfort is chair yoga.

Participants in one research did Yoga for two months. Researchers discovered that the yoga-practicing group's cortisol levels were lower than the control groups. The stress hormone cortisol might hurt your health if your levels are too high.

Additionally, Yoga's emphasis on breathwork aids in coping with and managing discomfort. Additionally, chair yoga practitioners may continue to wear their regular business attire, saving them the time and, perhaps more crucially, the embarrassment of seeing their boss dressed in Lulu lemons.

Chapter 3: Getting Started with Chair Yoga

You only require a chair, a little space, and a few minutes daily to practice chair yoga and walking. There are many different ways that you can begin practicing Yoga at a degree that is more appropriate for the requirements of your body and the objectives that you have set for yourself. And we still receive all the wonderful health benefits of the space. When we hear "yoga," many of us immediately picture toned and muscular bodies striking balance positions atop lofty mountains. In other phrases, Yoga has always appeared to be beyond our reach and has a mystique surrounding it. Please take comfort in the fact that the depictions here are not typical. It takes the pain of a lot of endurance, training, and determination to accomplish those yoga goals. It is extremely beneficial to both one's physical and emotional well-being.

Yoga is a gentle way to stimulate the body by building strength, releasing, and improving flexibility. Even though Yoga is typically a slow practice, finding poses, maintaining your weight, and working the musculature is a fantastic way to get your heart rate up without needing to run. You won't need much of it because it's efficient with space. You may still practice Yoga at home, particularly chair yoga, even if you don't have a lot of room to work with. You only need enough space to spread your arms in front of you and to either side without touching anything else. A calming atmosphere and a lack of noise are both desirable qualities in this location. Many people are looking for ways the exercise without having to leave the convenience of their homes in this ever-evolving world, particularly during this time of restrictive diets and worries about their health. One of the several fundamental forms of exercise that may be performed at home is chair yoga. You only need a chair and a little room to move around. You can set your speed or practice. Unlike visiting a class, practicing chair yoga in your home lets you go at an intensity you are familiar with. Also, you can tailor the exercises to a certain order of moves or concentrate on just one aspect, such as developing core strength.

3.1: Home Yoga Studio

Creating a home yoga class requires some preparation but also extraordinarily little effort. Establishing an environment that allows you to relax so you may utilize your meditation skills more effectively is crucial. A yoga studio should feel pleasant and serene. You ought to arrange it to reflect your unique aesthetic and spiritual needs.

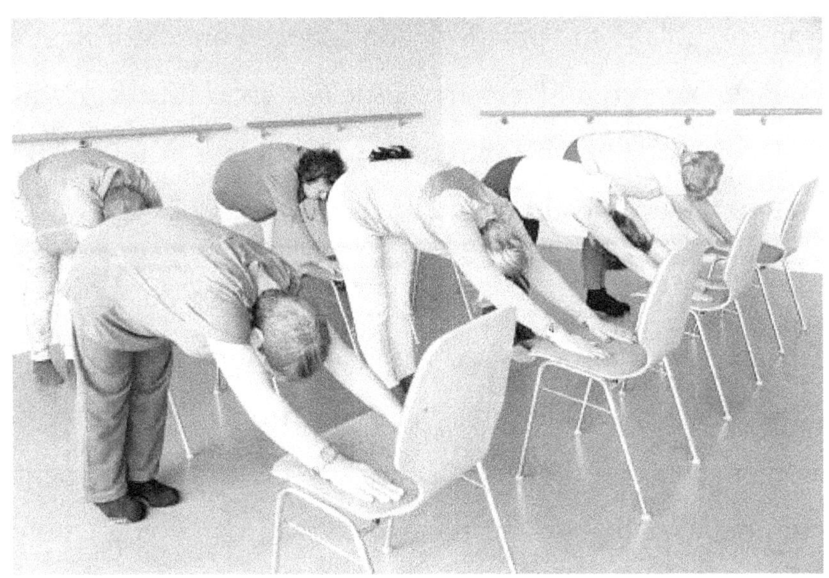

1. Designate Space

Determine a spot in your home where you can practice frequently and settle down there. Ensure you only use the area for yoga, meditation, and mindfulness practices. It doesn't matter if it's a room in your household or a distinct studio space; make sure you won't use it for anything else. This could be an unused bedroom, a portion of the main room, or any area of your property that is now sitting empty. A space of approximately 20 square feet is recommended as a decent starting location for a personal yoga studio. This will provide you with a comfortable space to perform your asanas. Check that there is sufficient space for you to move around while performing your sun prayers and to keep your yoga equipment. Plan to practice handstands and additional inversions. You should ensure sufficient space surrounding you, so you won't break anything if you collapse or fall. Other inversions include headstands and shoulder stands.

2. Have Purpose

The ideal setting for a yoga session is serene and soothing. You want to design an environment that encourages calmness, awareness, concentration, and focus on the present moment. Spend time visualizing your dream space and how you would react inside it. You should jot down one to five concrete things that you'd love to accomplish as a function of having a beautiful yoga studio and use those as the guiding principle when choosing design choices for the space.

3. Color Scheme

Your yoga practice should have a vibe that aligns with your intentions, and the colors you select should reflect that. For instance, if you desire to unwind, you might choose soothing colors such as blues and greens for your space. You might want to choose more vibrant colors like red colors and yellows if they want to give you a boost of energy. No matter what your objective is, you should always make sure all the colors you choose are complementary to one another. Your wall should be painted in subdued, warmer whites or cooler tones. These colors fade away rather than drawing attention to themselves. You can complement it with bolder and more brilliant colors with small household items or props.

4. Lighting

The way the room is lit has a significant bearing on how we feel. Too bright light can give people headaches and migraines and make them tired. On the other hand, a color temperature and brightness that is exactly right can make people feel more alert, creative, and focused. The natural light that has been filtered is going to be the best option, but if the area has narrow openings or you perform at night, you will need some additional light sources. Consider installing a dimmer button or buying lamps with 3-way controls to control how much illumination we get inside our homes. Dynamic practices like vinyasa or ashtanga should have warmer lighting, whereas relaxing styles like soft-to-the-touch yin and healing work better without dim lighting. Candles and lamps made from salt are fantastic choices for low-level illumination that induce a meditative mood.

5. Inspiration

The concept behind this one is straightforward: find something beautiful that can serve as a source of inspiration for you, whether it be a painting, sculpture, or photograph. This could be everything from a work of art to a picture of a close friend, mentor, or even a member of one's own family. It makes no difference what it is; all you need to do is look at it and consider why it makes your heart so happy.

6. Fragrances

To consecrate your at-home yoga area, start by lighting a fragrant candle, lighting a burning stick, or even simply spritzing oneself with essential oils. Avoid overdoing it since too much flame or smoke might harm your respiration. Carefully choose what you'll use as each perfume has various effects on us. Some people favor sweet aromas, while others enjoy pungent smells. Explore until you find what works best for you.

7. Maintain Cleanliness

Being with plants and tending them in any way cultivates attention, calm, and peace of mind. Plants also help clean the air in your back, especially during pranayama and difficult sequences. Go for flowers that thrive well with the sunshine in your environment. If you don't have a blue thumb, consider succulent plants, cacti, snake plants, plants with spiders, and ferns because they require minimal water.

8. Reflectors

A full-sized mirror is a terrific addition to any yoga school or home practice room. A big one will help you view yourself properly, giving them a better understanding of your symmetry. You will experience increased self-awareness and confidence as you move through your postures.

9. Décor

Candles assist in generating a soothing mood for relaxing and asana training. Purchase high-quality lamps that are dripless & smokeless. Try using organic soy candles because they burn more cleanly than paraffin wax. If you have apprehension about burning anything while using them, pick flameless lamps with LED lights.

10. Sound System

Music can boost your Yoga or meditative practice. Choose a sound that stimulates you and calms you. The music used for meditation is typically quite calming and serene, but many different song styles can also help you relax and unwind. Whatever the size of your room, a Bluetooth speaker that is either tiny or medium in size should work simply fine to provide an adequate amount of volume for practicing.

11. Crystals

In Yoga and meditation, crystals and stones impact the practitioner's mood, concentration, and energy. There are many sorts of rocks, each one having its specific features. These all have distinct applications, ranging from medicine to protection to cleansing. They also enhance your objectives and make wonderful additions to any personal practice room.

12. Statues

Monuments of Buddhas and other Hindu deities, such as Krishna or Ganesha, carved from stone, wood, or metal, can serve as a source of encouragement for your practice. You are free to position them wherever you like within your yoga space. The presence of statues might serve as an analogy for the goals we have set for ourselves. You can use them as a gentle reminder to focus on the here and now, concentrate on breathing, establish a connection with your power, and extend your heart.

13. Scared Alter

The altar is a wonderful method to gather all the necessary components for your practice to succeed. It is a place that you make for yourself to think about your life and the things that you hope to accomplish in the years to come as you go forward.

To begin, designate a space where you can display objects such as candles, incense, crystals, sculptures, photographs, and any other items that have meaning for you concerning your spiritual path. You might want to ensure that each of nature's five components is portrayed. Ensure that whatever you include there is significant to you somehow.

14. Furnish

Although you don't need much material to practice Yoga, you will need several essential yoga products to get the most out of your sessions. You will plan to spend a yoga mat, a few yoga blocks, and a yoga rope. A ball, meditation padding, a chair, a yoga ring set, and a resistance band are some additional things you should consider purchasing. Put your things away on a low shelf or inside a large basket so they are simple to get to but remain out of sight. This will give you the best of all worlds.

15. Organization

Each time you return to your practice environment, it should evoke feelings of novelty and freshness. After each session, make it a habit to put the decorations away and clear up the area before moving on to the next one. Be sure to clean the site regularly, including the mat and any other props you use.

Chapter 4: How to Use This Book

You may successfully use "Chair Yoga for Wellness and Wellbeing" with the assistance of this chapter. Your learning experience will be improved, and you'll get the most out of the information if you comprehend the book's organization, structure, and recommended reading sequence.

4.1: Overview of the Book

The book is divided into two parts, each with several chapters discussing various facets of chair yoga.

Section 1: Chair Yoga Benefits and Introduction

This section thoroughly overviews chair yoga, covering its description, roots in history, and particular advantages. It also instructs you on how to begin practicing chair yoga, emphasizing the need to create a proper environment, select the appropriate chair and devices, and take safety precautions. This section concludes with a training schedule that explains how to include chair yoga in your daily practice.

Section 2: Pose Guidelines and Daily 10-Minute Routine

This part emphasizes chair yoga's practical applications and offers thorough directions, step-by-step demonstrations, and variants for numerous postures and activities.

4.2: Guidelines for Effective Content Navigation

Consider the following advice to get the most out of what you learned and efficiently traverse the book:

- Check out the introduction: Reading the beginning of the book first will give you an understanding of its goals and subject matter. You will have a solid foundation and context from this for the next chapters.

- Depending on your requirements and interests, you may read the sections chronologically from beginning to end or concentrate on a few chapters that appeal to you. Each chapter may be read alone and is intended to be self-contained.

- Consider Making Notes and Reflecting: As you read the chapters, consider making notes and reflecting on the important ideas, suggestions, and insights. You'll be able to customize your practice and increase your comprehension.

4.3: Usage and Proposed Reading Sequence

Although your tastes and requirements may change the proposed reading sequence, we advise using the following strategy:

1. Start with Chapter 1 first: Read Chapter 1, which introduces the idea of Yoga in chairs, its history, and its antecedents.

After reading this chapter, you will have a strong basis for comprehending chair yoga's foundational ideas.

2. Look into Chapter 2: Continue reading Chapter 2, which explores the advantages of chair yoga. Learn about its distinct advantages for certain demographics and its mental, physical, and emotional benefits. Knowing these advantages will encourage and drive you while you practice chair yoga.

3. Explore Chapter 3: Chapter 3 discusses how to begin practicing chair yoga. Learn how to set up a proper environment, choose the appropriate chair and devices, and ensure safety by making changes. Pay close attention to the value of proper breathing methods since they are essential to practicing chair yoga.

4. Chapter 5: Personalize Your Practice Go to Chapter 5 to obtain a recommended chair yoga training schedule. This chapter outlines the weekly exercises, development, adaptations, and integration of meditation and mindfulness practices. Utilize this plan as a template to modify it to suit your unique demands and objectives.

5. Explore Section 2, which contains Chapters 6, 7, and 8, and embrace the practical aspects. These chapters provide comprehensive directions, step-by-step drawings, and

variants for various stances and exercises. While doing chair yoga, you may use these sections as a resource, concentrating on the fundamental postures, advanced modifications, and your 10-minute daily program offered in Chapter 10.

Remember that you may change this recommended reading sequence to suit your choices and requirements. The idea is to provide the tools to fully use the information and tailor your chair yoga routine to improve your well-being.

You will thoroughly grasp chair yoga, including being prepared to start a joyful path of health and well-being by paying attention to the navigation suggestions and the recommended reading sequence.

Chapter 5: A Training Plan to Start with Chair Yoga

Planning for Yoga is effective. Here are some exercises for you to try if you are starting.

5.1: Plan for Seniors to Practice Chair Yoga Once a Week

The great practice of chair yoga is an excellent way to increase flexibility, strength, and relaxation while catering to senior citizens' requirements and capabilities. This five-day schedule for chair yoga is tailored to the rare needs of older citizens. Always pay attention to what your body tells you and alter the poses to fit your comfort level.

Day 1: A Slow Start to Get Warmed Up

Beginning with the Chair Cat-Cow Stretch can help you increase flexibility while gradually warming up your spine. Carry out five cycles of cat-cow breathing while moving in time with your breath. Urdhva Hastasana, also known as Chair Pose with Raised Hands, is the next pose you should do to stretch and lengthen the upper body. Take a concentrated breath and increase your arms toward the ceiling while keeping a decent posture. Uttanasana, also known as Chair Forward Bend, should be used as the final pose to help release tension in the back and hamstrings. Exhale, bend forward as much as possible, bringing your hands to rest on the ground if feasible. Take a deep breath in, and then raise your arms back up. It should be repeated a few times.

Day 2: Turns and Maintaining Balance

To stretch and strengthen the side body, start with Chair's Extended Side Angle (Utthita Parsvakonasana). After coming into a forward fold, reach your left hand back and place your fingertips on the outside of your left foot. Next, twist to the right to open your chest. Maintain this position briefly, then switch sides and do it again. Move to Chair Pigeon to improve your flexibility and open up your hips. Hold this position for a few deep breaths with your right ankle crossed over your left thigh. Repeat the process with your left leg. Finish with Garudasana, also known as Chair Eagle Pose, to improve your balance and stretch your shoulders. If possible, you should try to cross your accurate thigh over your left thigh. Bring the palms of both hands together while traveling your left arm over your right arm at the elbow. Switch sides and repeat the exercise after holding for three to five breaths.

Day 3: Flowing While Seated

Start with Chair Spinal Twist (Ardha Matsyendrasana) to improve spinal mobility and digestion. This pose is also known as Chair Spinal Twist. Place yourself on the chair so that you are facing the left side of the room, then twist to the left while holding on to the back. Take a deep snort to lengthen the spine and let the breath out to turn. On the other side, repeat the process. Move into Chair Warrior I, Virabhadrasana I, to develop your strength and stability. Keep the right leg in posture over the area of the chair while you swing the put leg behind you. Raise your arms to the ceiling, maintaining a strong stance. Flow into Chair Warrior II (Virabhadrasana II) to open the hips and strengthen the legs. Open your arms with the right arm coming forward and the left going back. Turn the torso to the left and gaze out over the right fingertips.

Day 4: Deep Stretch and Relaxation

Begin with Chair Forward Bend (Uttanasana) to release tension in the back and hamstrings. Exhale and fold forward, letting your hands rest on the floor if possible. Take a deep breath in, and then raise your arms back up. It should be repeated a few times. Move into Chair Pigeon to open the hips and stretch the glutes. Hold for a few breaths. Finish with Final Relaxation:

Chair Savasana. Sit with your eyes closed and hands in your lap, allowing your body to absorb the benefits of the practice. Take a few minutes to relax and transition into the rest of your day. Remember to breathe deeply and listen to your body throughout the procedure. Chair yoga offers a safe and accessible alternative for seniors to experience the myriad benefits of Yoga while sitting comfortably on a chair. Enjoy your weekly chair yoga plan and feel the positive effects on your body, mind, and spirit.

5.2: Chair Yoga and Mindfulness

Traditional Yoga has been adapted to be practiced in chair yoga, where the participant either sits on the chair or uses it for support while performing the poses. People who have trouble moving around or are otherwise unable to participate in standard Yoga can derive significant benefits from this style of practice. Yoga in a chair has been demonstrated to lower stress through several important methods, each of which will be examined in greater depth.

1. Relaxation Response's Activation

Chair yoga requires you to engage in exercises in deep breathing, which are one of the key components in inducing the relaxation response within the body. The physiological response following stress, sometimes known as the "fight or flight" response, is the opposite of this reaction. Your body enters a state of peace and relaxation due to the relaxation response, which causes your heart rate to reduce, your blood pressure to drop, and the tension in your muscles to release.

2. Happy-Making Hormones

Endorphin, serotonin, and oxytocin are the hormones responsible for causing emotions of joy, contentment, and relaxation. Chair yoga is known to enhance the release of these chemicals. Chair yoga helps prevent the adverse effects of stress chemicals such as adrenaline and cor by raising hormones that make people happy. When you get home from an extended period at work, try these 12 yoga poses you can do in your office chair.

3. Enhanced Capacity to Connect the Mind and Body

Chair yoga fortifies the bond between one's mental and physical selves via slow, controlled movement and gentle stretching. Because of this increased awareness, practitioners can better recognize and cope with the sources of stress, ultimately reducing their overall stress levels.

4. Improved Capacity for Self-Direction and Independence

The ability of practitioners of chair yoga to successfully perform poses and practices that they may not have considered feasible is one of the ways that chair yoga helps create self-efficacy. This sense of achievement plus empowerment contributes to enhanced confidence and a more optimistic outlook, both of which can assist in lessening the stress levels that an individual is experiencing.

Section 2: Pose Instructions and 10-Minute Daily Routine

Chapter 6: Chair Yoga Poses and Exercises For Beginners

Warm-ups are crucial while doing chair yoga. Any physical activity that involves introductions improves performance and reduces the risk of injury. Warm-ups for chair yoga are brief, so don't neglect them. The blood supply to muscles rises to 75% after a few warm-up exercises.

Yoga routines often begin with warm-ups known as vinyasa flows or sun salutations. Vinyasa is a term for synchronizing breath with movement. We may set our minds in the right frame to flow and move more easily by saluting the sun by swinging the body with the breath.

Warm-up exercises might be compared to movement meditations. We often go through our days aimlessly. Our bodies and minds are in harmony when we take the time to connect our respiration to our activity, and we get a lot more positive attitude on the day. Additionally, we begin to conduct our lives with greater clarity and purpose. It's astonishing to believe that a few simple conscious actions may have such a significant impact, but they can!

6.1: Sitting Warm-Up

1: Any Version of Virasana (the Hero Pose), 1 to 5 minutes

If your thighs, knees, and hips can handle it, this is my go-to meditation posture. It's also a terrific place to start a sitting practice. Please do Sukhasana (Easy position) instead if this position hurts your hips, knees, or legs.

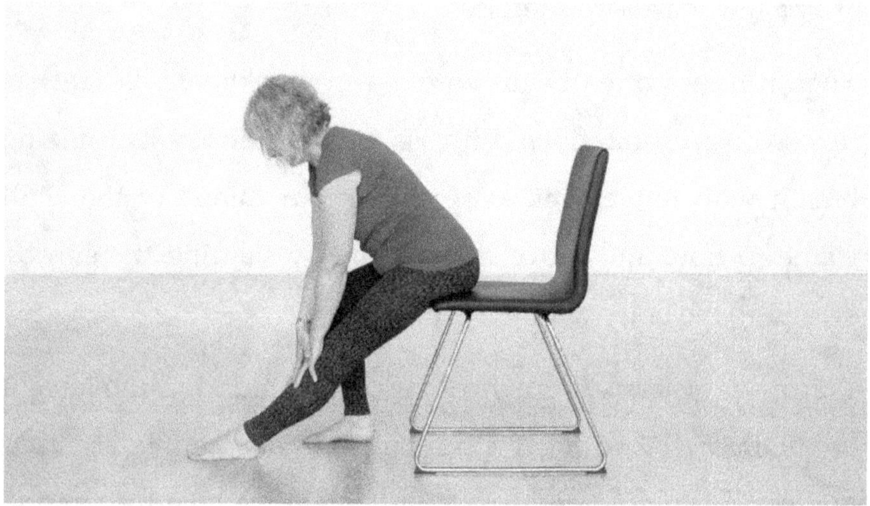

Enter into whatever variation of Hero Pose permits you to sit in a neutral curve in the middle of your back and is comfortable for you.

From here, spend some time being grounded by paying attention to how your entire being feels as you begin your practice and how your respiration is moving. Set an objective for the duration of your exercise if you choose.

2: Six rounds of Marjarasana (Cat-Cow) Pose while seated

Doing the cat-cow is a gentle technique for exercising your hip and spine joints.

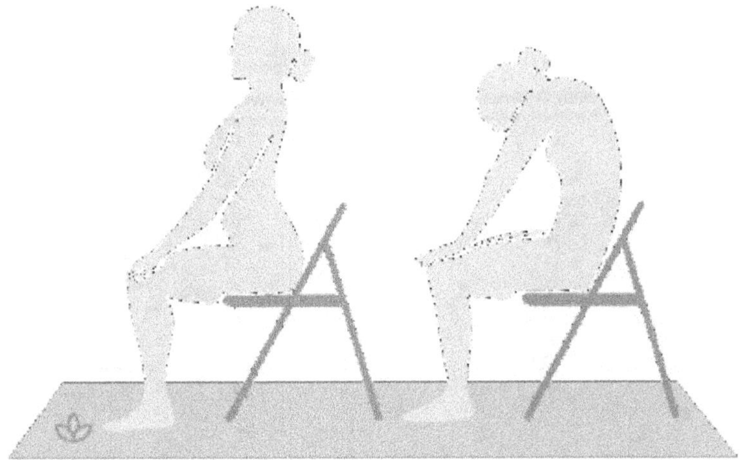

Do six repetitions of Cat-Cow while standing in Hero Position (not sitting in a chair), as illustrated above, swaying your hips and spine with your breathing. In Sukhasana, you may do Cat-Cow if Virasana isn't ineffective.

3: 30 to 60 seconds, twice, Arms Overhead Pose

Urdva Hastasana, also known as the "Arms Overhead Pose," is a fantastic posture for strengthening and stretching the upper back, arms, and forearms. The bound variation of the pose also extends your wrists and forearms.

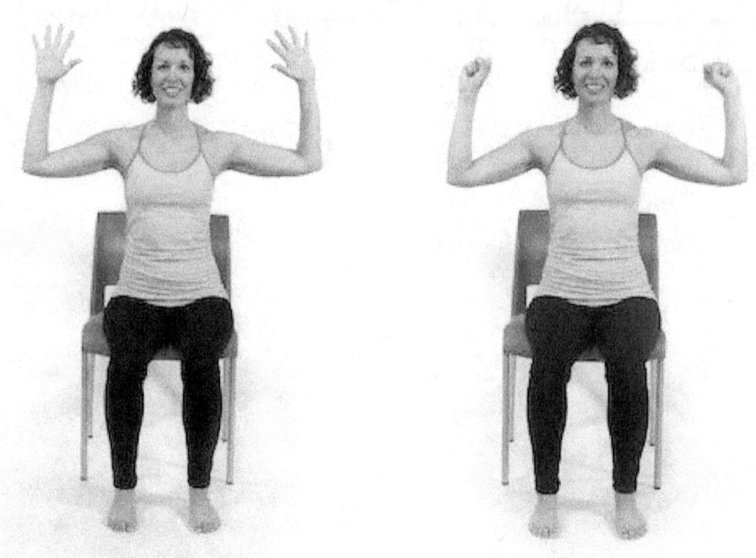

1. When you inhale, sweep your upper body alongside your eardrums while interlacing your fingers and pushing both hands toward the ceiling.

2. Exhale after thirty to sixty seconds, then let your arms go.

3. Alternate the direction of your finger crosses, then repeat for the same duration on the second side.

4. Once you have completed all variations of Hero Pose (and Easy Pose), lean forward, and take a few breaths on your hands and knees. Extend one leg back to stretch the ankle and calf region while keeping your toes on the ground. Repeat with the other leg.

4: Easy Seated Side Bend with Dynamic to Static

This position elongates your arms, ribs, and waist on the sides. Enter into any Easy Pose variation that seems comfortable for you to begin. If your pelvis is pushed back and the back of your spine is rounded, put some folded towels under the hips to raise them.

Start by mastering this pose's dynamic variation:

1. The right shin should be in front while you sit in Easy Pose. A folded blanket should be placed under your hips to enable you to sit comfortably with a relaxed, erect posture.

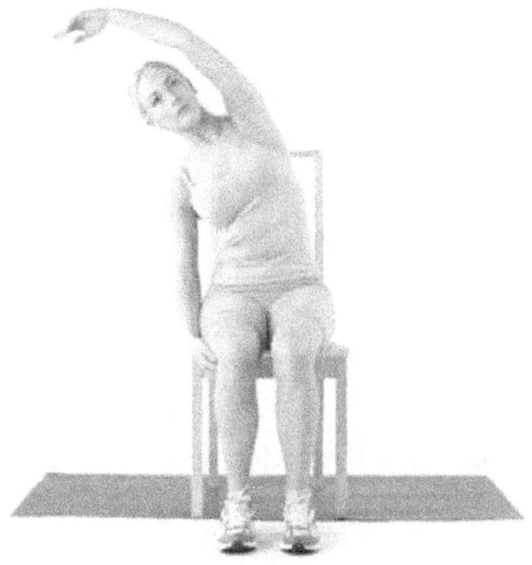

2. Put your fingers a couple of inches from the outer edges of your hips on the ground.

3. Straighten your arms out from the sides as you inhale, then as you breathe out, bend them to the right and place the palm of your hand on the ground.

4. Return towards the center when you take a breath. Touch the ground with your fingers on the outer edges of your hips. One round only.

5. Bend to your left as you exhale, then return to the center as you inhale.

6. Then, as you exhale, incline your right body. Return to your core and bring your fingers back down to the floor on an inhale. You are now in the second phase.

7. Repeat the procedure with your left leg in front after a couple more rounds.

8. After that, hold the posture still for 30 seconds off each side.

9. With your right foot in front, bend your right side into a side angle with your left arm extending over and up to your right and the palm of your right hand touching the floor approximately 6–12 inches from your hips. Your torso should also be somewhat bent to the right.

10. Return to your upright position after 30 seconds, then repeat a side bend towards the left while moving your left leg to the front.

5: Upward Plank Pose, 30 to 60 seconds

This sitting backbend helps expand your chest, making it helpful for other sitting poses, standing presents, and more. It also serves as a nice warm-up for backbends if you practice them.

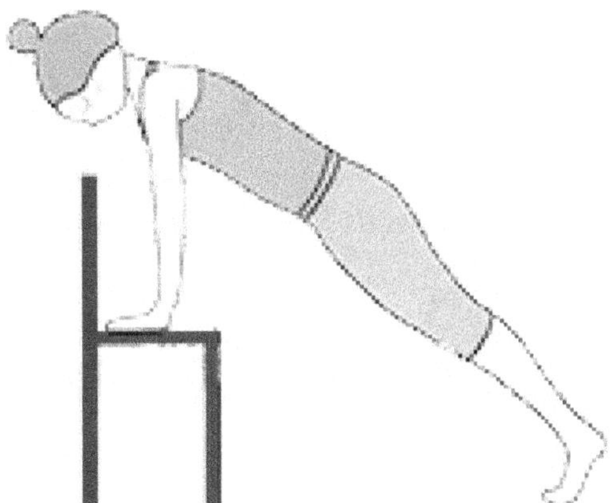

6: Static to Dynamic: Simple Sitting Twist

This position is a great method to give your spine some rotational action, which enhances spinal flexibility, strength, and range of motion.

Come into Easy Pose to begin. Next, do six rounds of the energetic variation of the Easy Sitting Twist:

1. Exhale while turning to the right, then inhale while bending back to the center. When you exhale, turn to the left and back to the center when you inhale. One round only.

2. Two times back and forth while keeping time with your breathing.

3. On the exhale, first, move to the left; on the inhale, move back to the center; finally, go to the right; and so on.

4. After that, hold a static Easy Seated Twist, slowly shifting to the right and towards the left.

5. 30 to 60 seconds, twice, Easy Sitting Pose

The hip and spine joints will become more mobile and flexible in this posture, reducing stiffness.

Come into the posture by placing your right knee ahead of your left. Remain for 30 to 60 seconds. After that, place your left leg in front of the right, and assume the stance again for 30 to 60 seconds.

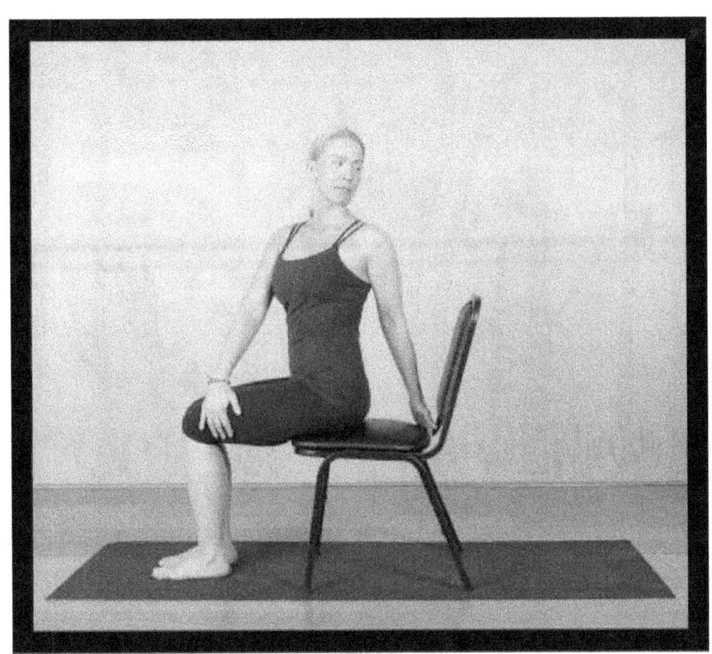

8: 30 seconds in Boat Pose, three times

Your front leg muscles and core muscles get stronger in this posture.

This variation is suitable for brand-new practitioners learning the posture for the first time, for individuals who are unfit or recuperating from a medical condition that has left them exhausted, or for those with balance problems. It is also an excellent place to start for individuals with back issues, as it is gentler on the back.

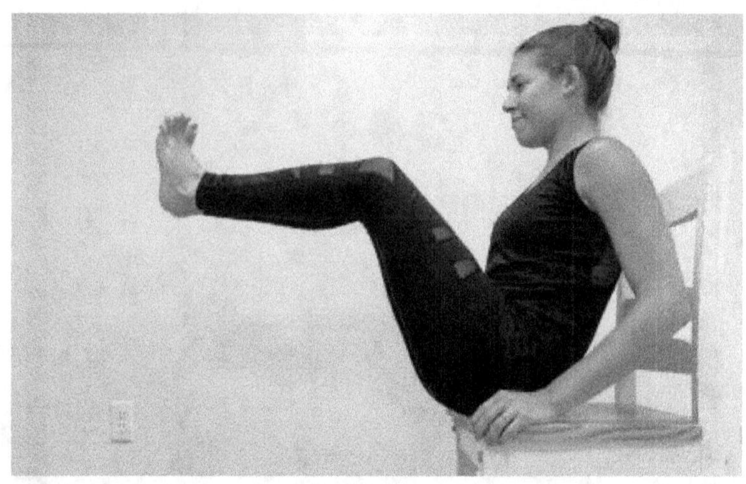

1. Beginning on the floor with your feet flat and knees bent. Alongside your hips, place both of your hands on the ground.

2. You should now walk with your arms about a foot or two behind you, extending your elbows slightly backward as you do so. You should also tilt your body around 30-45 degrees while maintaining a balanced head position over your shoulders.

3. Swing your heels up to the floor in a parallel position as you exhale, maintaining your legs straight together or slightly apart.

4. Stay for six to eight breaths. You may eventually work up to remaining for one minute as your stamina increases over time.

5. Move your hands forward as you raise your chest vertically while bending your knees and lowering your feet to the floor to exit the posture.

6. Repeat, as necessary.

Before moving on to the remainder of your exercise, extend your legs outwards on the floor, then roll them from side to side.

6.2: Chair Yoga Pose While Standing

6.2.1: Branch Pose

A standing pose improves balance and strengthens the ankles and legs. Modifying the chair partially eliminates the balancing component, allowing our students to feel anchored and concentrate more on the pose's hip "opening" impact.

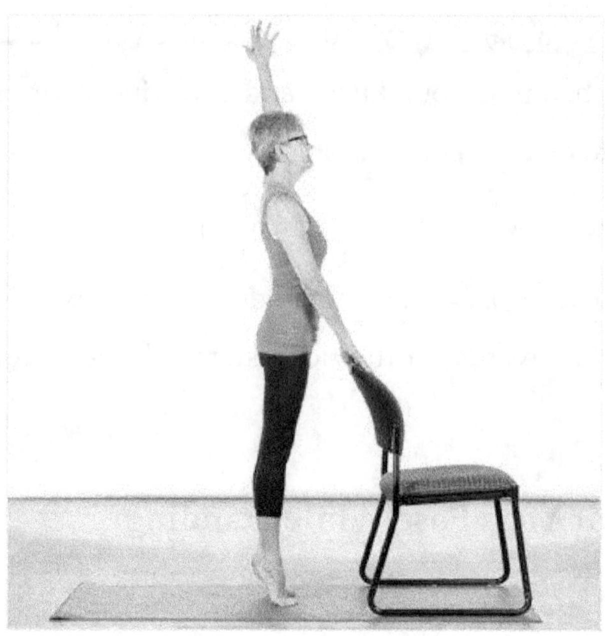

1. Face the chair and place your hands on the frame without your feet hip-width apart.

2. Position the heel of your right foot upon the inside of your left thigh or calf, depending on what feels secure and comfortable.

3. To maintain stability and balance, engage your core.

4. Raise your arms in the air or place your hands in a prayer posture at the center of your chest.

5. Hold the position for a few breaths while maintaining balance and paying attention to your breath.

6. Continue on the opposite side.

6.2.2: Warrior Pose

Another balance position with legs facing opposite directions tests the hips and pelvis.

While utilizing the chair, we may concentrate more on pelvic stability by removing the balance component from the position.

When performed dynamically (from mountain position to warrior 3 using a chair), this posture may empower certain persons who have previously fallen.

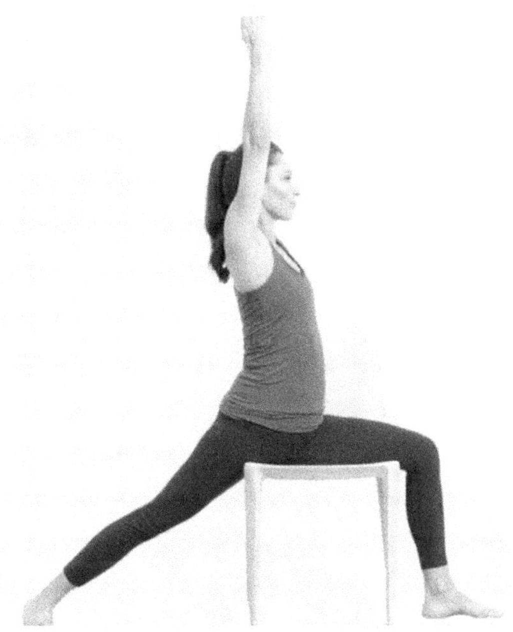

1. Stand around the chair and support yourself by resting your hands against the back.

2. Lift the right leg full back, and parallel tighten your abdominal muscles.

3. Maintain a square posture with the chair.

4. Extend your arms straight back beyond you or forward.

5. Concentrate on balance and alignment while you hold the position for a few breaths.

6. Continue on the opposite side.

6.2.3: Voluntary Triangle

Suppose the hamstring or abduction flexibility is lacking. In that case, this asana might seem quite risky since the muscles in our legs are actively stabilizing as we rotate.

By modifying the position using the chair, we may concentrate more on turning while keeping our balance and the spine's neutral alignment.

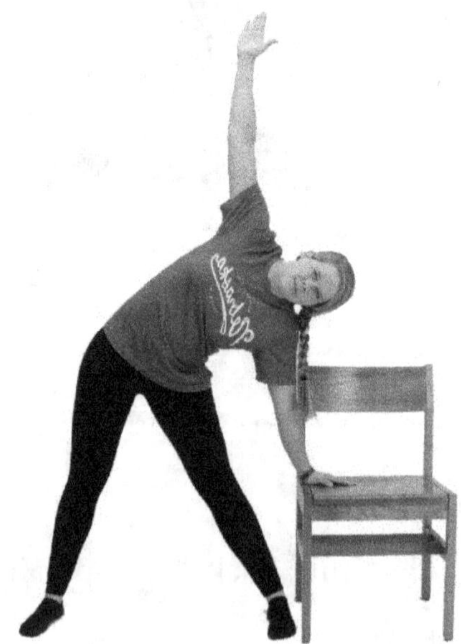

1. Face the chair while standing with your toes wider than hip-width apart.

2. For support, rest your left hand against the back or seat of the chair.

3. Turn your torso towards the right while reaching up with your right arm.

4. Maintain a long spine and twist from the waist.

5. If it's convenient, gaze up toward the palm of your hand.

6. Maintain balance and feel the twist as you hold the position for a few breaths.

7. Continue on the opposite side.

6.2.4: Moon Half Floating

A challenging balancing stance that needs your front body to be open for you to get its full advantages.

When in perfect alignment, it seems your body supports you since all the endocrine system glands are lined up in this stance.

We may enjoy the full benefits of this position and feel good by working with a chair or a wall.

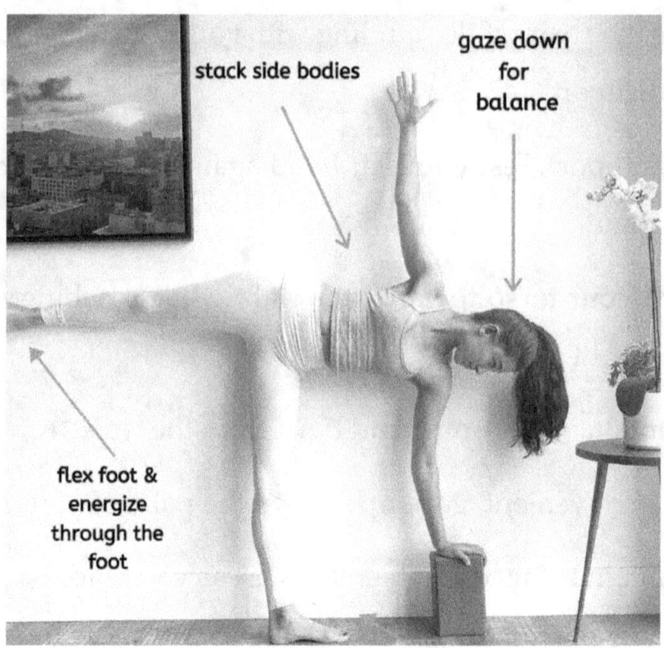

1. Stand close to the seat and support yourself by resting the palm of your hand on the back or middle.

2. Lift the leg on your right off the floor and stretch it out to the opposite side while you shift your weight to your left leg.

3. Maintain a forward-facing posture with stacked hips and shoulders.

4. Look at your left hand while raising your left arm toward the ceiling.

5. Remain in the position for a few inhalations, noticing the opening in your front body.

6. Continue on the opposite side.

6.2.5: Leader Pose

This position, often known as a squat, is excellent for developing the legs, but individuals with limited mobility frequently cannot stoop low enough to properly benefit from it.

The chair variation of this stance gives the pupil security. The exercise can be even more dynamic, ranging from a sit-to-stand position to a low hovering over a chair to a squat towards the end.

Since the arm posture heavily depends on flexibility in the shoulders and latissimus dorsi power, cactus hands could be more advantageous.

1. With your feet hip-width apart, stand directly in front of a chair.

2. Sit into a chair by lowering your hips backward until your glutes contact the bottom of the seat.

3. Keep your spine straight and your knees in line with your toes.

4. Raise your arms upward or forward while lifting your chest.

5. Hold the position for a few breaths, focusing on engaging your core and feeling the power in your legs.

6. Get back up to your feet and stand.

6.2.6: Lunge

This position lengthens the hip flexors and extends your thighs and groin. A difficult stance for many.

A certain amount of hip mobility and equilibrium is necessary for the posture, which also involves a slight backbend to maintain the spine extended and get the full benefits of the position.

The chair meets all those requirements, which also helps with balance and reduces the need to stretch the spine forward.

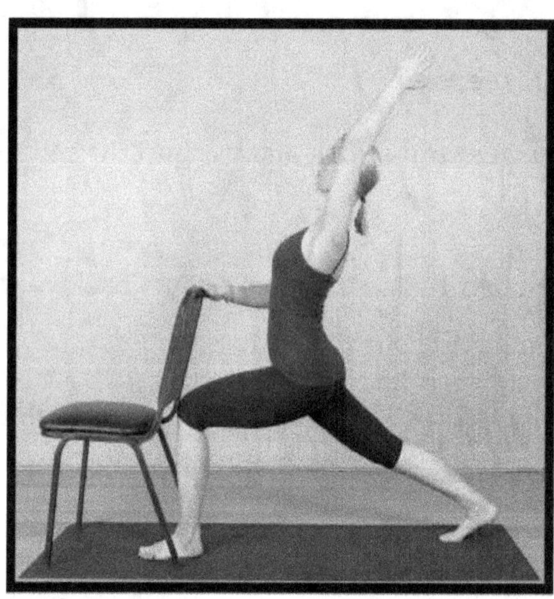

1. Stand beside the chair and support yourself by resting your hands against the back.

2. Lunge forward while stepping your right leg forward and maintaining your right knee in line with your ankle.

3. Maintain a straight back leg and plant the heel firmly on the floor.

4. Feel a little stretch in the upper part of your left hip as you lengthen your back and elevate your chest.

5. Maintain the position for a few breaths, emphasizing flexibility and balance.

6. Continue on the opposite side.

Chapter 7: Advance Chair Yoga Poses For Seniors

You could think that you cannot practice Yoga as you are unsteady on your feet, suffer from persistent discomfort, have poor balance, or have trouble getting out of your seat, but you could be completely wrong. People who suffer from chronic pain or disability or don't feel sufficiently centered to practice Yoga on their own may find that chair yoga is a more suitable and less risky alternative. Drawing into soft stretches, known to reduce stress, can help alleviate some of the worry caused by persistent pain and impairment. If we can reduce some aspects of the stress, we can alter how the patient experiences the pain.

Pain that persists and the emotional misery associated with it never allow your body or brain to rest. This is the vicious cycle of pain. We may erase a few of the anxiety and possibly even ease some of the pain in our lives if we bring awareness and pleasure to some of the mental tension we hold onto. Sometimes as we become older, we experience a loss of confidence in ourselves. We are worried that we will injure ourselves and aren't sure if we have the strength to progress through the poses. We use the chair as our starting point for standing postures, or we can even change standing poses into sitting poses when we practice chair Yoga. When we have a sense of safety and security, we care less about getting hurt and instead direct our attention to the parts of our bodies attempting to feel better.

The concept underlying chair yoga is the same. While seated in a chair, Yoga can provide many of the same health benefits as performing a complete yoga routine. The goal is to maintain the same level of awareness and breathing throughout the practice; we are modifying the postures to make ourselves feel more at ease. Many medical professionals will recommend that you keep your inactive muscles active. The breathing exercise expands your lung capacity and flushes toxins out of your lungs, two benefits medical professionals typically cite as reasons to recommend the practice. You can benefit greatly from your routine even if you only focus on your breathing and mindfulness practices. When you combine this method with some little stretching, you will feel the tension leaving your body. We don't understand how much our muscles tighten when we keep mental or physical stress. Suppose we can let go, even just a little bit. In that case, we may be rewarded with fewer negative emotions, a lighter body, increased self-assurance, and possibly even some relief from our physical discomfort. Bringing oneself into the here and now lets you feel sensations.

Put your shoulders down and relax them while you stretch your spine as much as is comfortable. Just close the retina and focus on your breathing. Block out everything else on your to-do list, including all the places you must. Just give yourself some time to relax and regroup right now. Allow your breath to move through your body and into your skeletal system. Bring your attention to how your body is feeling right now. Pay attention to your body's feelings, but don't criticize or become upset. Instead, be mindful of which body parts feel beneficial and which portions may not. Now, take a deep breath and allow that new breath to fill the upper part of your body with air, much like a balloon. Also, let all that air be from your lungs as you exhale. Take three long, deep breaths while you do so. Relax and maintain regular breathing as you focus on how each breath makes your body feel. You've just engaged in some mindful practice. It can be summed up like that. You should breathe into the moderate stretches as you move into them.

You can unwind and take pleasure in the feelings that come from moving while being supported by the chair. Because of the attention, you can be conscious of how any stretch feels to your muscles, enabling you to alter the space to suit your needs. Chair yoga confers all the health advantages of a standard yoga session without the associated risks. You can practice chair yoga at some yoga studios, as well as in a variety of community and senior centers. Inform your instructor of any ailments you may be experiencing so they can guide you through safe adaptations of some positions. Regular chair yoga can instill self-assurance, relieve stress, and help build strength and energy. Allow another person to give you those things. You deserve it! Check with your physician and see if a seated yoga class is in your area.

7.1: Advanced Chair Yoga Techniques For Seniors

7.1.1: Neck and Shoulders

Because it is a mild form of stretching that can help develop flexibility, strength, and balance, chair yoga is an excellent type of seated Yoga that senior citizens can do. Because they release pain, stress, and exhaustion from the neck and upper back muscles, the neck and shoulder strains are among the quickest and most helpful poses for seniors to perform while seated in a chair during a chair yoga session. The following is a list of some basic seated yoga poses that could be done by senior citizens in only a few minutes. Ensure you are seated upright with your feet firmly planted on the ground. Take a deep breath, bring your shoulders up toward your ears, and then let out your breath as you roll your shoulders back down. Perform this action multiple times, ensuring a slow and controlled pace throughout.

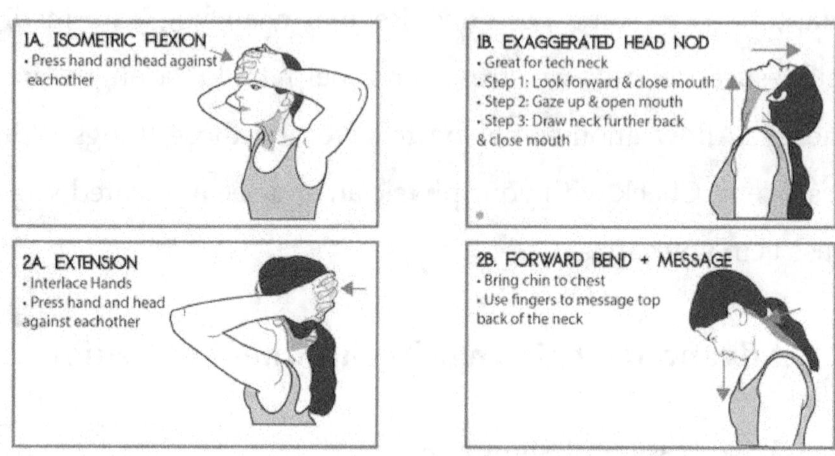

Start by firmly placing your feet on the ground and sitting straight in your chair for seated neck rolls. Take a deep breath, tuck your chin towards the center of your body, and slowly roll your head from side to side while maintaining a downward stare. Exhale, repeat the process multiple times while keeping calm and controlled movement.

Cat-Cow Stretch While Seated To begin this stretch, sit up straight in your favorite chair with the soles of your feet planted firmly on the ground. Take a deep breath and round your back as you drop your head and shoulders and lift your chin to face the ceiling. Exhale, round your back by bringing your chin closer to your chest and thrust your shoulders forward as you round your back. Perform this action multiple times, ensuring a slow and controlled pace throughout. These simple stretches for the neck and shoulders are wonderful for folks who are just starting with sitting Yoga for seniors because they are easy to perform. Flexibility can be improved with chair yoga, Poses Done While Seated Forward Folding and Twisting. As we get older, our flexibility may naturally decline. Chair yoga is a great approach for seniors to enhance their flexibility in a way that is easy on the body and works well for more sedentary people. Chair yoga postures such as seated downward fold and twist provide moderate to deep stretching and encourage good posture. Both of these poses are simple to practice.

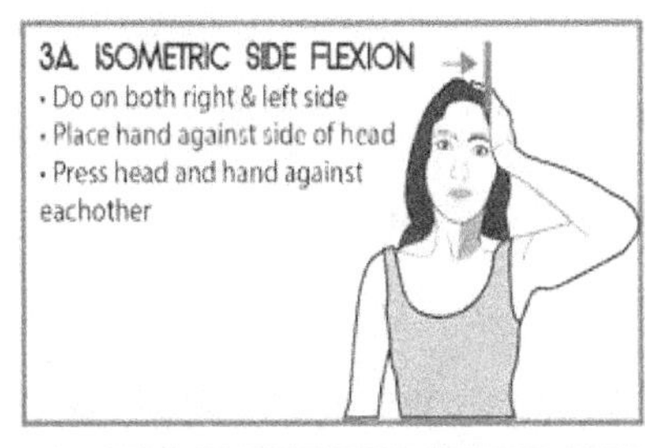

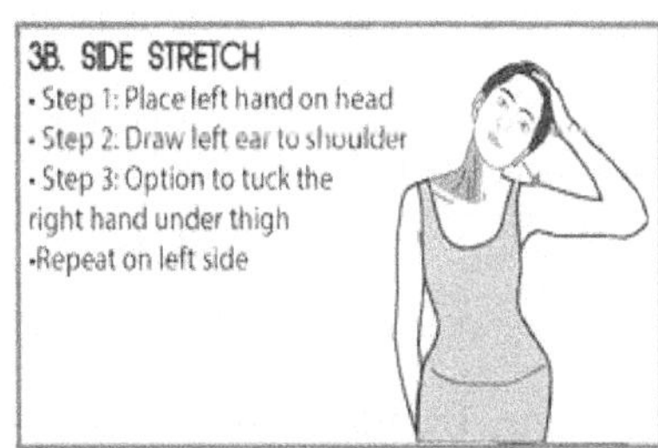

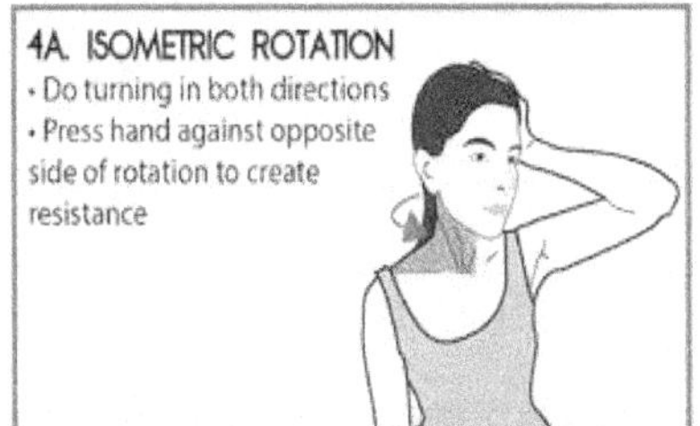

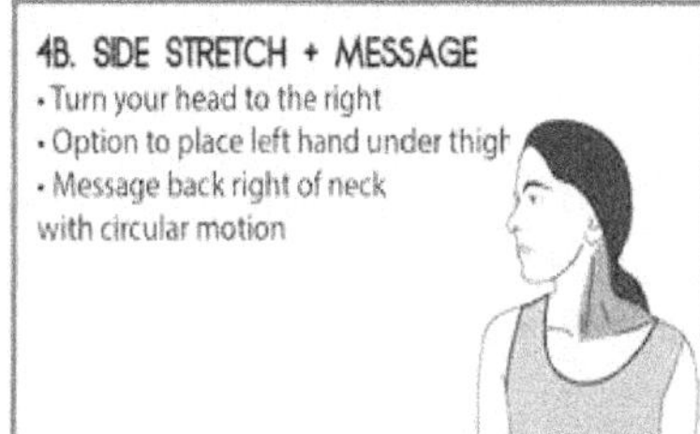

One of the most effective ways to stretch the shoulders and back is to perform a seated forward fold. To assume this position, begin by installing with your back in a neutral position, your legs extended in the direction toward you, and your feet placed about hip-width apart. Take a few deep breaths, and as you're doing so, lean forward from the waist until your hands are almost touching the ground. While you breathe in and out and hold the posture for a few seconds, keep the natural curve in your spine. Exhale completely, then go into a seated position and slowly rise to your feet. The abdominal muscles, the thighs, and the spine can be worked on effectively through seated twist postures. Choose a chair and place your feet firmly on the ground about shoulder-width apart. Your right hand should be placed on the rear portion of the chair, and your left hand should be placed on the outer edge of your right knee. Turn your body to the right in a slow and gentle motion while keeping your neck and shoulders relaxed. After holding the position for a while, taking several deep breaths, release it and repeat it on the other side.

7.1.2: Flexibility

As we get older, our flexibility may naturally decline. Chair yoga is a great approach for seniors to enhance their flexibility in a way that is easy on the body and works well for more sedentary people. Chair yoga postures such as seated downward fold and twist provide moderate to deep stretching and encourage good posture. Both of these poses are simple to practice.

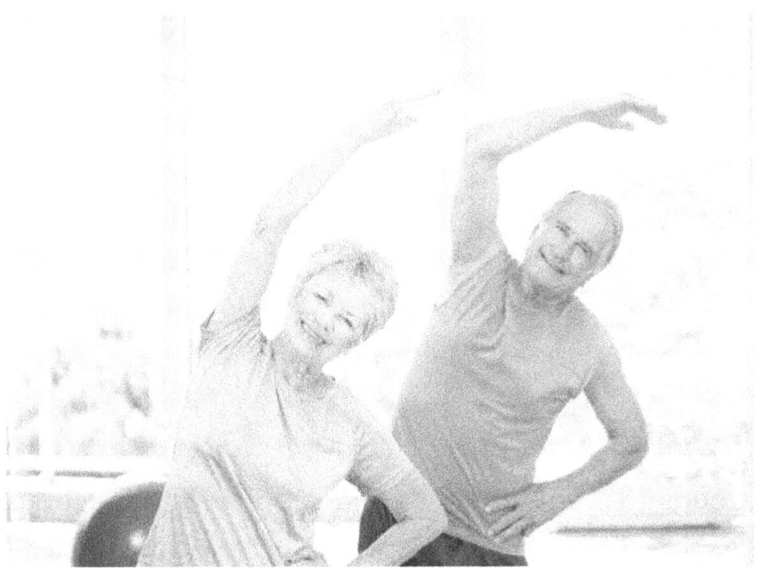

A seated forward fold is one of the most effective ways to stretch your shoulders and back. To assume this position, begin by sitting on your back in a neutral position, your legs extended in the direction toward you, and your feet placed about hip-width apart.

Take a few deep breaths, and as you're doing so, lean down from the waist until your hands are almost touching the ground. While you breathe in and out and hold this position for a few seconds, keep the natural curve in your spine. Exhale completely, then go into a seated place and slowly rise to your feet.

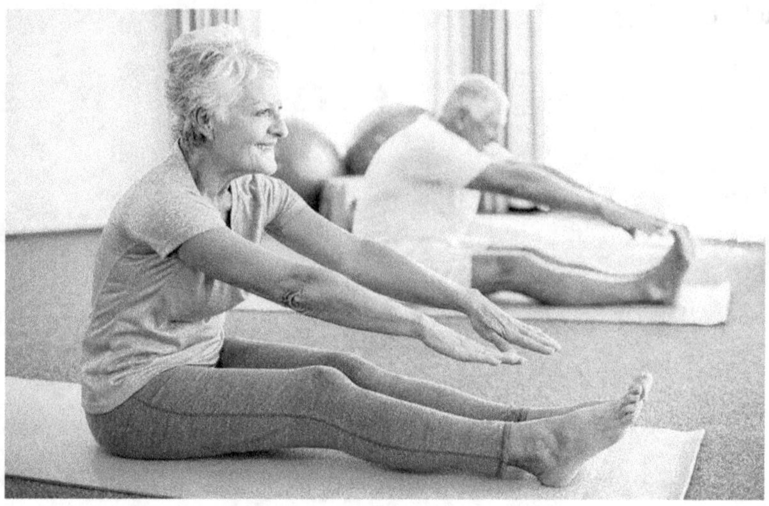

The abdominal muscles, thighs, and spine can be worked on effectively through seated twist postures. Choose a chair and place your feet firmly on the ground about shoulder-width apart. Your right hand should be placed on the chair's backrest, and your left should be placed outside your right knee.

Turn your body to the right in a slow and gentle motion while keeping your upper body relaxed. After holding the position while taking several deep breaths, release it and repeat it on the other side.

7.1.3: Strength Training

For seniors looking to increase their strength and overall physical fitness, chair yoga is a fantastic activity. The sitting warrior or chair pose variations give mild chair yoga to seniors and sat Yoga for novices, which can assist in toning muscles, developing balance, and enhancing energy levels. Chair yoga is also beneficial for the elderly. Warrior postures performed while seated are excellent for developing strength in the upper body and the abdominal and back muscles. To get started, move to the very edge of the seat and plant both of your feet squarely on the ground. Put your hands on the chair's armrests and lift yourself until you are in a position where you are halfway between sitting and standing, with your knee joint bent at a ninety-degree angle and your forearms fully extended. Return to the beginning position after holding this position for a little while. You can take this posture to a more difficult level by leaning forward from the waist just a little bit, maintaining a straight line with your legs, and pressing your hips back just a little bit. Ensure your arms are fully extended while maintaining the stance for several seconds.

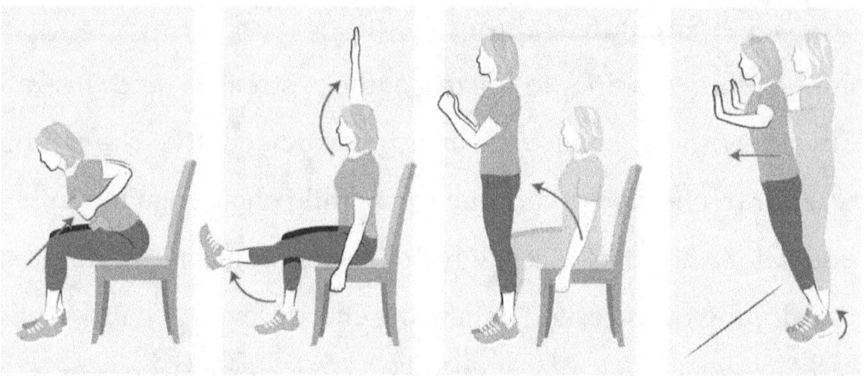

Chair postures can build strength across the arms and abdominal region. To get started, adjust your posture to sit up tall on the chair with both feet firmly planted on the ground.

Put your hands on the chair seat with your fingers pointed toward your feet, then press down on them to slightly raise yourself off the chair seat. When you hold the stance for a few seconds, be sure that your back is straight, your chest is up, and your shoulders are down.

Holding onto the rear portion of the seat while elevating your bottom off the heart & extending your limbs out in the direction of you until they are parallel to the ground is an advanced variation of this position. Keeping this pose for some seconds before returning to the initial appointment.

These mild chair yoga postures for seniors & seated yoga positions for beginners will assist in increasing the body's flexibility, strength, and balance. Seniors who engage in consistent practice can experience improvements in their mobility, posture, and overall well-being.

7.1.4: Balance Training

Because they improve one's balance and overall body awareness, the balancing poses part of chair yoga is essential to any practice. Asanas that focus on balance, such as the tree pose and the sitting half-moon pose, can be performed while seated, making them ideal for seniors who may have difficulties standing for extended periods. To begin, you will want to ensure that you are seated upright in your chair, with both feet planted firmly on the ground and your hands softly resting on top of your legs. Raise your right knee and place it under your left thigh while you inhale. Then release your breath. Maintaining your balance requires you to contract your muscles and press the sole of your foot firmly on your thigh.

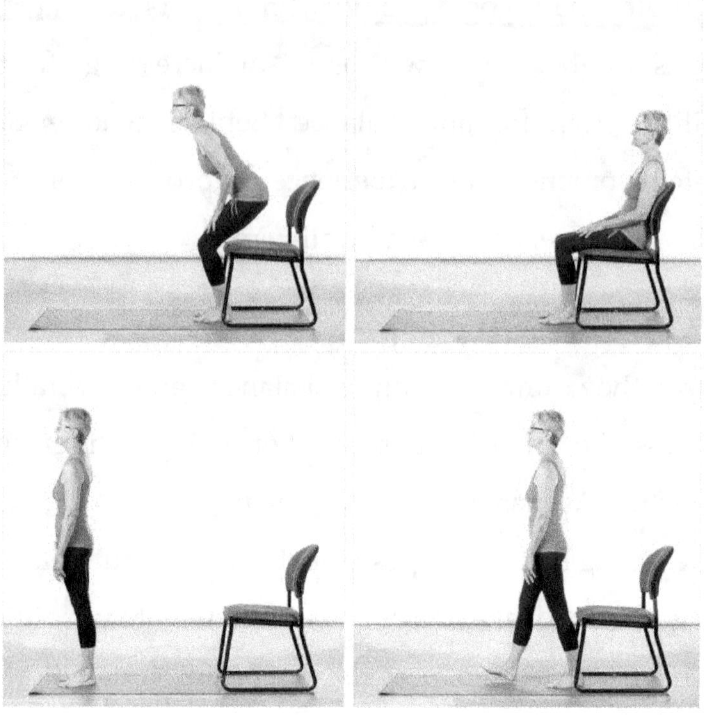

You can rest your hands on your hips or lift them behind your head to make the pose more difficult. After holding for five to ten breaths, switch sides and repeat.

The seated half-moon position is an excellent approach to increase the stability and power in the torso and the core. To begin, adjust your seat perpendicular to the floor and flex your abdominal muscles. While you do so, position your right hand such that it is outside of your right leg. At the same time, extend your left arm towards the side at the level of your shoulder.

Leaning your lower body to the right should be done while maintaining a straight spine and taking deep breaths. After you have held this position for five to ten breaths, switch sides and do it again.

These two postures complement any chair yoga practice but are particularly beneficial for seniors who want to enhance their balance. Begin cautiously and pay attention to any discomfort or pain you experience while practicing. These positions, when practiced daily, have the potential to enhance posture as well as power, balance, and flexibility.

7.1.5: Relaxation Poses

Senior chair yoga has been shown to have several positive effects. Mobility, harmony, and relaxation are all improved by chair yoga. In addition to easing tension and relieving exhaustion, it can help improve one's general well-being. Meditation and other practices that support the practitioner in calming their mind and body, such as breathing exercises, are also integral to chair yoga.

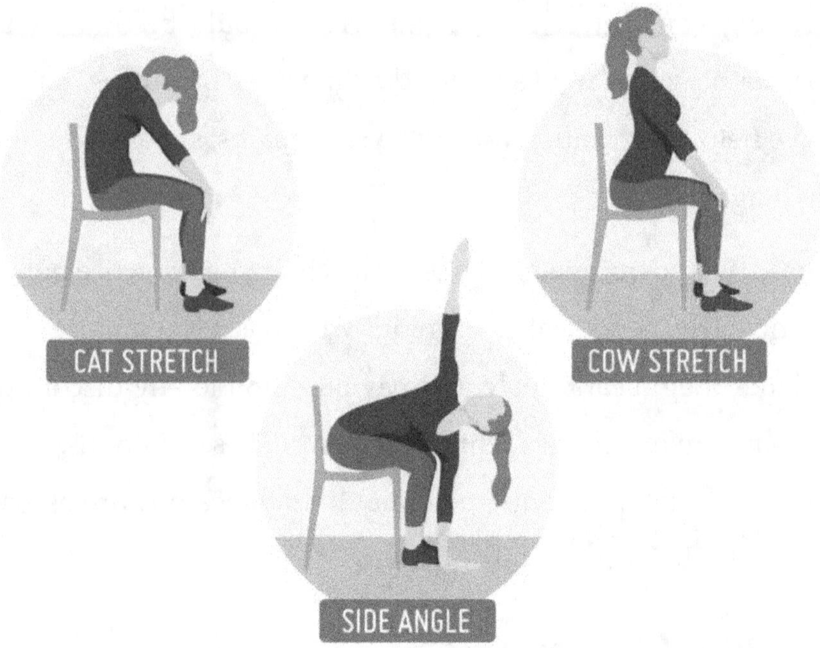

The mind and the body can both benefit greatly from practicing meditation. When practicing sitting meditation, one concentrates on the breath while seated in a chair. It may be beneficial to close one's eyes and concentrate on the feeling of breathing in and out via the nose. While focusing on one's breath can be an effective way to rid one's mind of other thoughts and make it possible for one's mind to become still and relaxed, this practice is not for everyone.

When combined with breathing exercises, chair yoga can produce an even deeper state of relaxation. Exercises focusing on breathing help slow breathing, lowering stress and bringing mental tranquility. To perform a basic breathing exercise, take a long, deep breath through the nose, hold it for a minute, and gently let it out through the mouth. It is possible to carry out this process multiple times until one feels completely relaxed.

The benefits of chair yoga can be maximized by incorporating the relaxation techniques mentioned in various sequences. A greatly beneficial practice for senior citizens can be created by combining several positions with meditation. Practiced regularly, chair yoga can assist in the reduction of physical pain, the promotion of mental clarity, and the enhancement of general well-being.

Chapter 8: Step-by-Step Instructions

Because we know how important it is for you to have direction and guidance during your practice, we will give you in-depth explanations that will assist you in completely embodying each posture.

These guidelines will act as a compass for you, guiding you toward correct alignment, thoughtful movement, and the development of inner calm, regardless of whether you have prior experience practicing yoga or are just starting. Chair yoga is an alternative to traditional yoga that is less strenuous and more approachable. It enables practitioners to get many advantages of yoga while sitting in a chair rather than on the floor.

You will gain the ability to begin on a path of self-discovery, good health, and mental clarity after reading these pages, which contain a wealth of information and insight that will equip you to do so. We are going to explore the connectivity of our bodies, minds, and breath as we practice the discipline of chair yoga. This will allow us to create a harmonic symphony of recovery and rejuvenation for ourselves.

We encourage you to create a presence throughout this practice by directing your attention to the sensations inside your body and fostering a profound connection with your breathing through each posture. You can reawaken latent energy, get relief from stress, and experience a revitalized feeling of vigor if you practice the discipline of mindful movement.

The thoughtfully prepared directions will lead you through an uninterrupted flow of postures, enabling you to flow elegantly from one position to the next as you go through the sequence. We advise you to constantly listen to the rumblings of your intuition and respect the particular requirements and constraints posed by your physical makeup, adjusting as required.

Establish a holy space around you as you immerse yourself in this chapter. A sanctuary is where you may engage yourselves in your practice of armchair yoga. Candles should be lit, soothing music should be played, and you should allow the ambiance to help cultivate a serene setting that will assist your path of self-care and self-discovery.

Therefore, let us go together on this life-altering journey of chair yoga. As we gently go through each posture, let us remember to recognize and appreciate our bodies, brains, and spirits while we do so. This chapter will motivate you, providing the resources and direction to develop a practice that will last a lifetime and feed you on every level.

The following is a detailed explanation of how to do each pose:

8.1: Cat-Cow Stretch

Do this stretch while seated on a chair without your feet planted firmly on the ground and your back in a neutral position.

- Put your hands on the bottoms of your legs or the top of your thighs, whatever is most comfortable for you.

- Cow posture requires you to inhale, round your back, and bring the upper body on your back while twisting your shoulders downward.

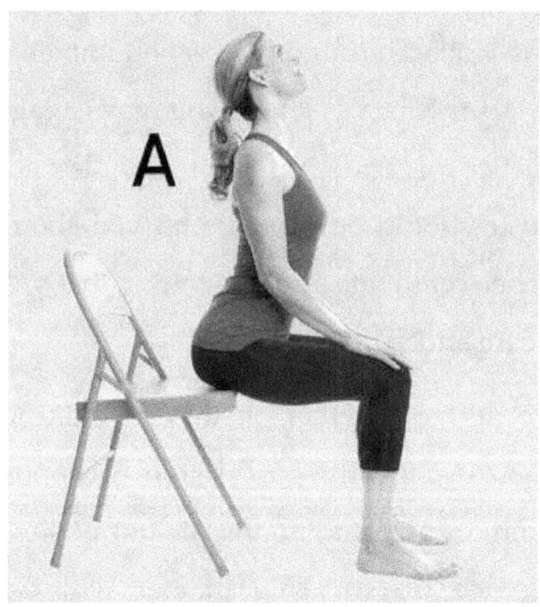

- While exhaling, round your back by pulling your shoulder or head forward and lowering your chin nearer your chest (this is the cat stance).

- Switch between the cow stance and the cat pose for the next five breaths, synchronizing the motions with your breath.

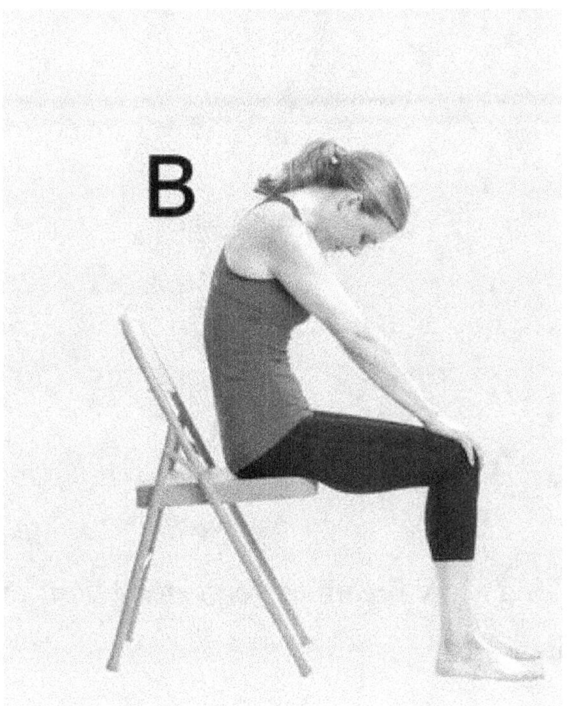

8.2: Urdhva Hastasana

- Sit on a chair having your feet planted firmly on the ground and your back in a neutral position.

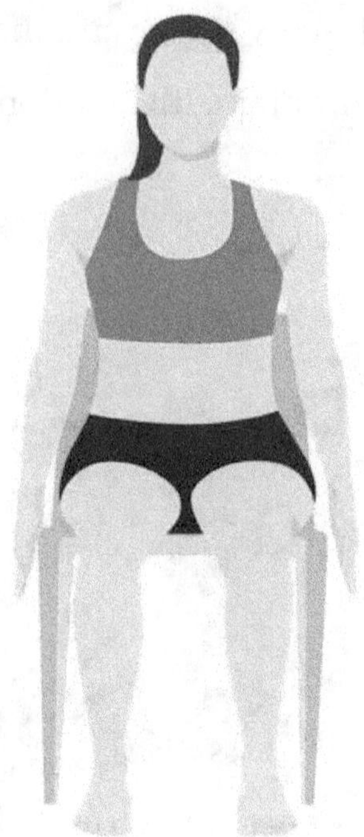

- Take a long, slow breath as you extend your arms toward the ceiling.

- Maintain a relaxed state in your shoulders while keeping your rib cage over your hips.

- Throughout the position, be sure to have a good posture in your upper body.

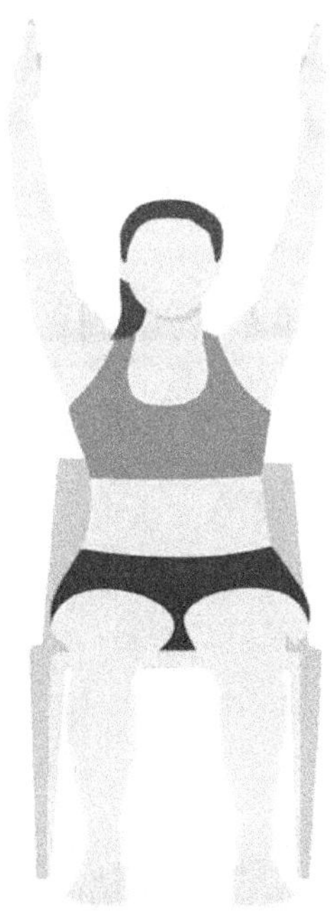

8.3: Chair Forward Bend

Exhale as you come backward over the legs into an upward bend while seated on a chair.

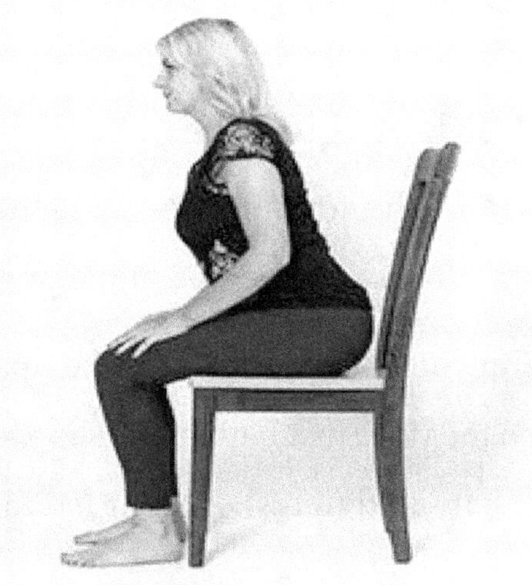

- Let your hands relax on the ground if they can reach the ground. In such cases, you should let them hang loosely or pull them down to your shins.

- Relax and let your head drop down low while you do so.

- Perform this movement a few times, coordinating it with your breathing each time.

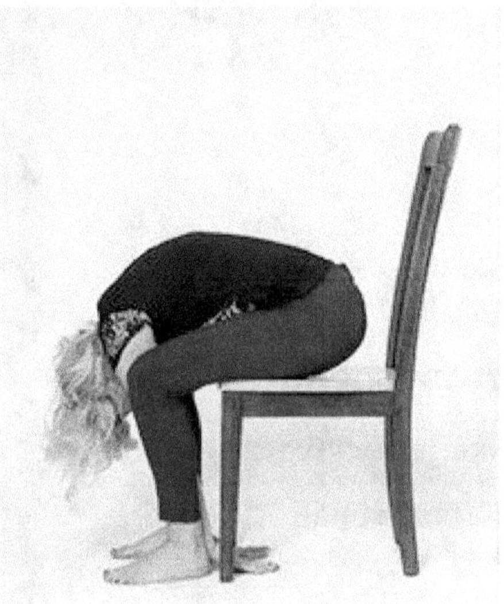

8.4: Extended Side Angle Pose

From the posture of the forward bend, maintain the folding position to get into the extended side angle pose.

- Either position your left hand so that the tips of your fingers are resting on the floor just beyond the border of the left foot or raise your left hand to rest on your left knee.

- Take a deep breath and rotate to the right while bringing your right arm above and gazing upward.

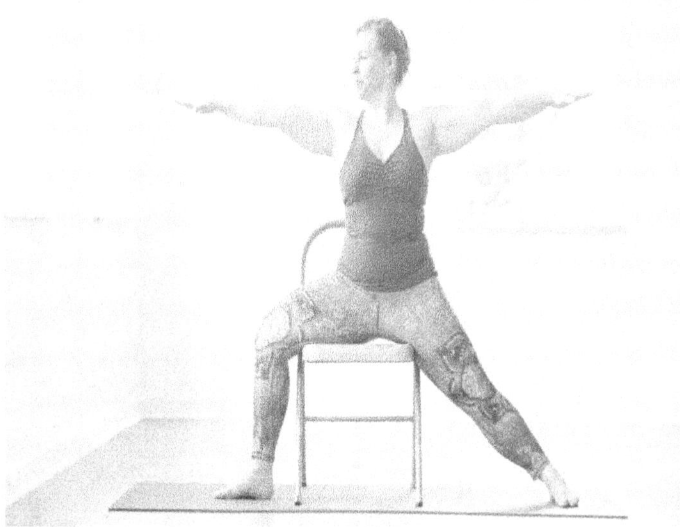

- Allow your chest to open while maintaining this stance for a few deep breaths.

- Pull your right hand down to rest by your side as you exhale.

- Continue holding the same posture but elevate your right arm and bring your left arm down.

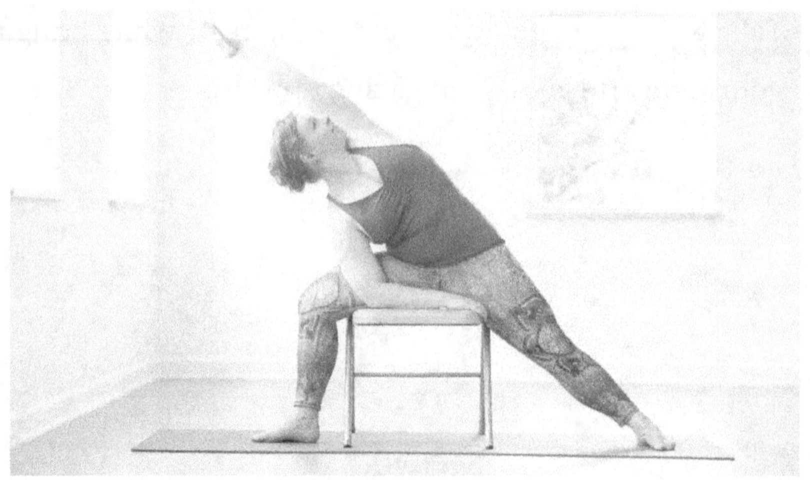

8.5: Chair Pigeon

While seated in an upright position on the chair, bring your right foot to rest upon your left thigh, forming the shape of figure four with your body.

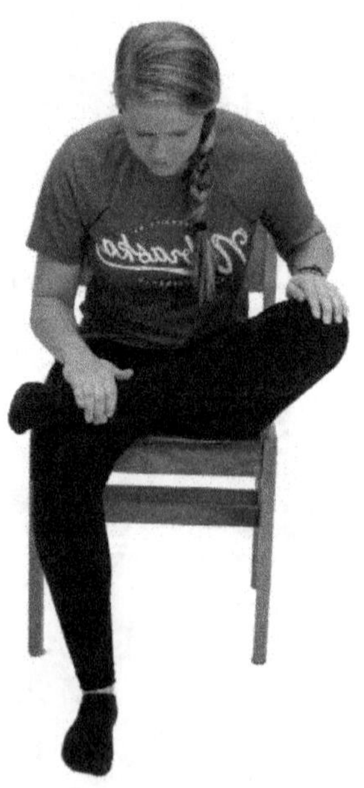

- Keep the angle that you have between the knee and your ankle.

- You should hold this posture for anywhere between three and five breaths.

- You might try leaning forward just a little bit to get a better stretch out of it.

- Now repeat the process with your left leg.

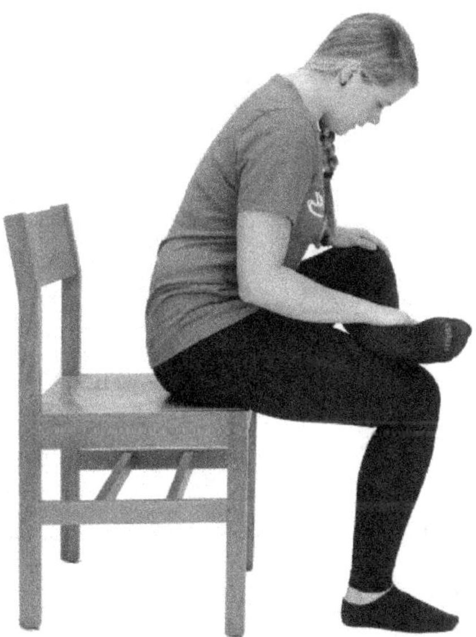

8.6: Chair Eagle

begin by sitting in an upright position on the chair. Next, cross your right leg over your left leg if feasible.

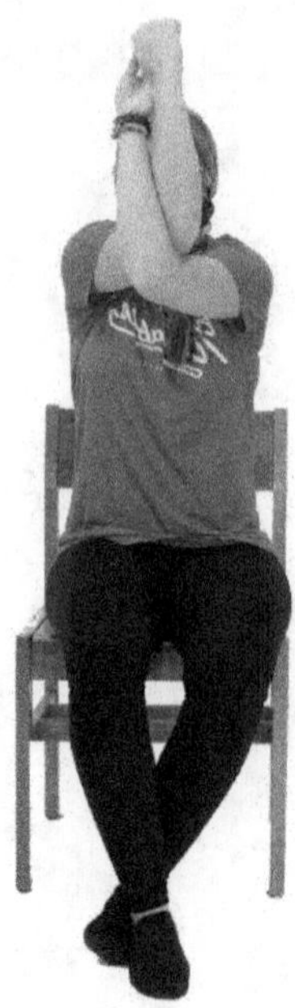

- Cross your arms around the elbows, ensuring your right arm is positioned over your left.

- Bend the elbows and try to bring the palms of your hands together as much as you can.

- Raise your elbows and move your shoulders toward your ears while maintaining a neutral spine position.

- Maintain this stance for anywhere between three and five breaths.

- Do the same thing on the opposite side.

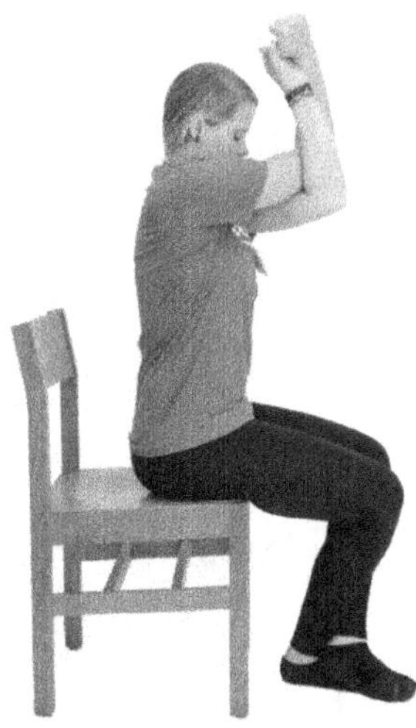

8.7: Chair Spinal Twist

Sit on the chair sideways, with your left side facing the chair.

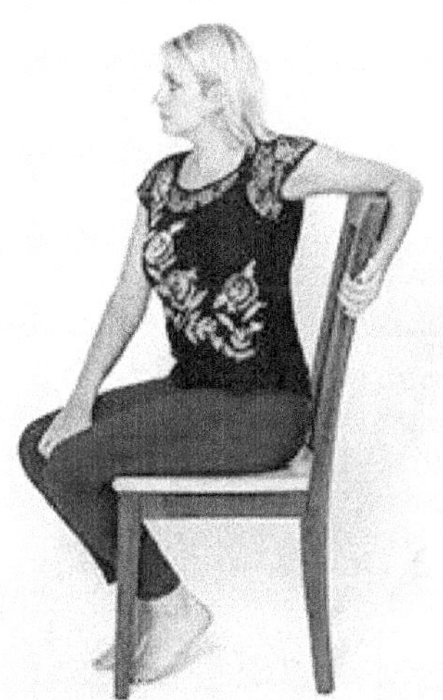

- For a twist that targets the spine, rotate your upper body to the left while extending your back onto the seat back of the chair.

- Maintain the twist until the count of five breaths.

- To do the twisting the other way, move your legs to the opposite side of the seat and repeat the exercise.

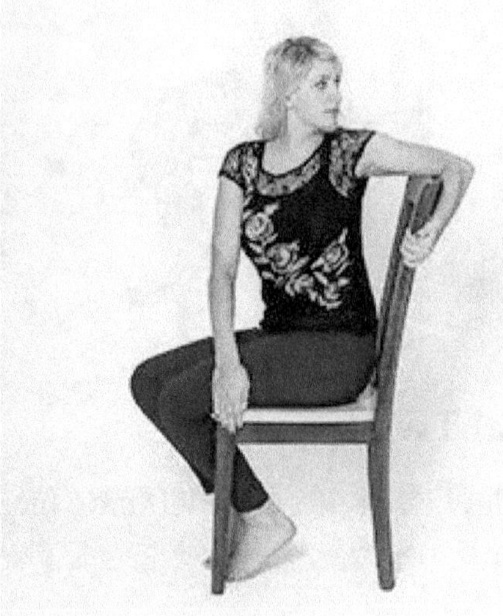

8.8: Chair Warrior I – Three Breaths

Sit on a chair and stretch your right leg out to the side.

- Swing the left leg across you and place the bottom of your left leg on the floor so that it is parallel to the chair seat.

- Put your left leg into a straight position.

- To get into Warrior, I posture, ensure your body is towards your proper leg while inhaling.

- Maintain this stance until the count of three breaths.

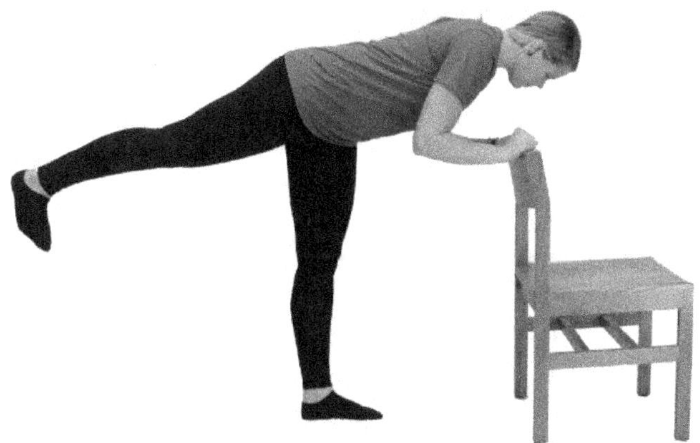

8.9: Chair Warrior II– Three Breaths

In the second variation of the Chair Warrior exercise, expand your arms by bringing your right arm forward and stretching your left arm back as you exhale.

- To align properly with the front edge of the chair, rotate your torso to the left and push your left hip backward.

- While maintaining the Warrior II stance for three breaths, turn your gaze outward over your right fingers.

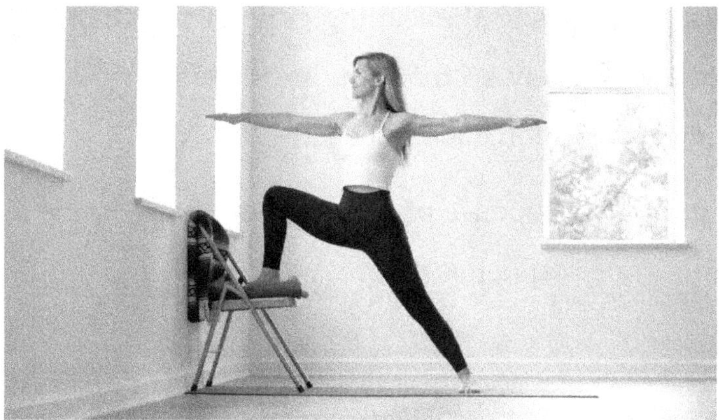

8.10: Reverse Warrior

As you inhale, let your left arm glide over your left leg. At the same time, elevate your right hand toward the sky. This will bring you into the Reverse Warrior stance.

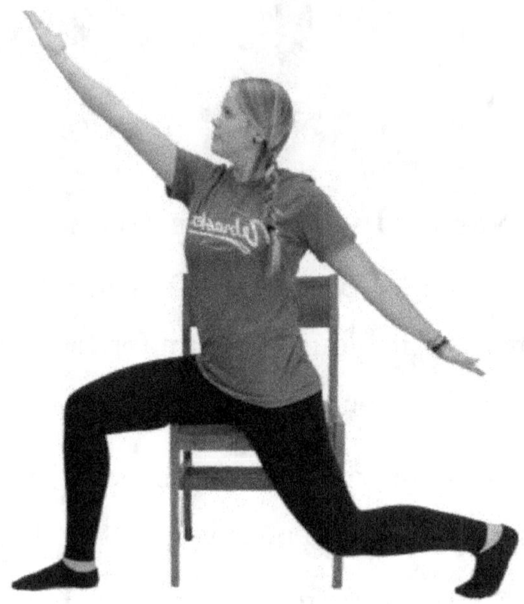

- Maintain this stance until the count of three breaths.

- Raise both legs to the leading edge of the chair, and then rotate your body so that you are seated on the chair in a sideways position, facing the left side.

- Perform the sequence of five warrior poses on the left side in the same manner as before.

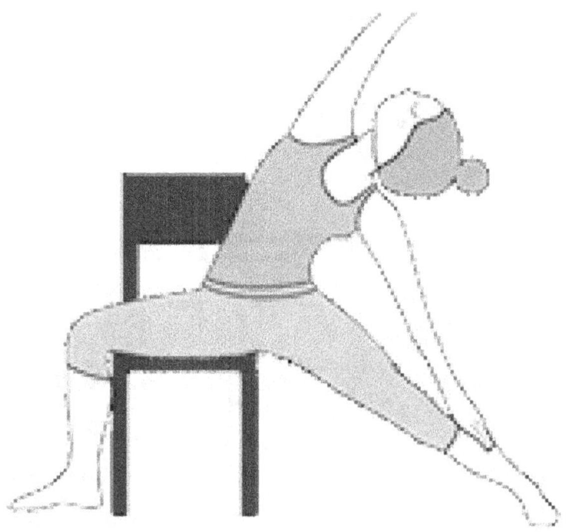

8.11: Chair Savasana

- Sit quietly on the chair without your eyes shut and your hands resting on your lap. This is the position for the Chair Savasana yoga pose.

- Unwind and give your body time to process the changes the exercise has brought about.

- Take a few moments to relax in this setting savasana before moving on to the next part of your day.

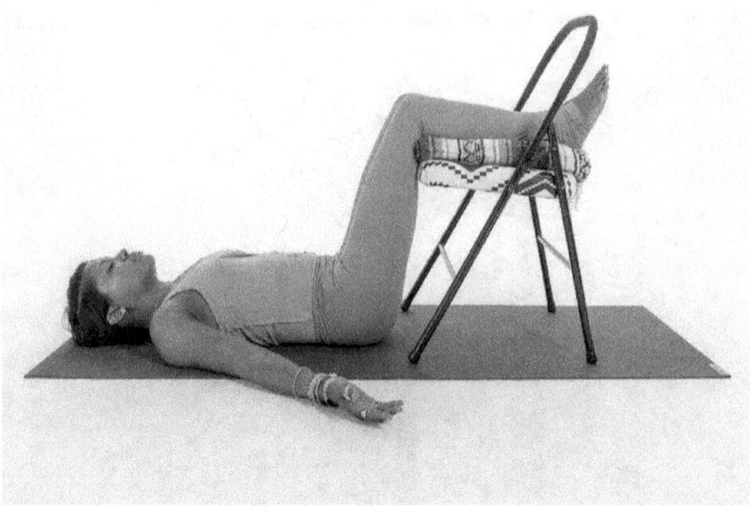

8.12: Mountain Seated

Simply focusing on your breath, checking in with your stance, and engaging your core are all fantastic things to do in this position. After striking each of the perspectives below, hit this one.

- Inhale deeply and sit upright straight, letting your spine lengthen.

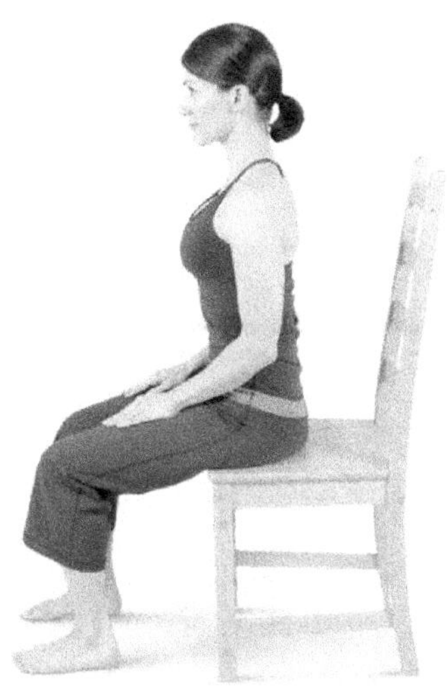

- Put your sit bones—the lowest section of your tailbone or the two bones that support your weight when you sit—into the chair as you exhale.

- Knees should be directly over ankles, and legs should sit at 90-degree angles. There should be some space between your knees. Normally, your fist should fit in the space between your knees. However, your bone structure could need more space.

- As you exhale, take a long breath, and relax your shoulders, resting your back, belly button toward your back, and arms down at the sides. If your chair includes armrests, then you may need to move them slightly forward or wider to allow for the armrests.

- Lift your toes and plant your feet firmly into each of the four corners to activate your legs.

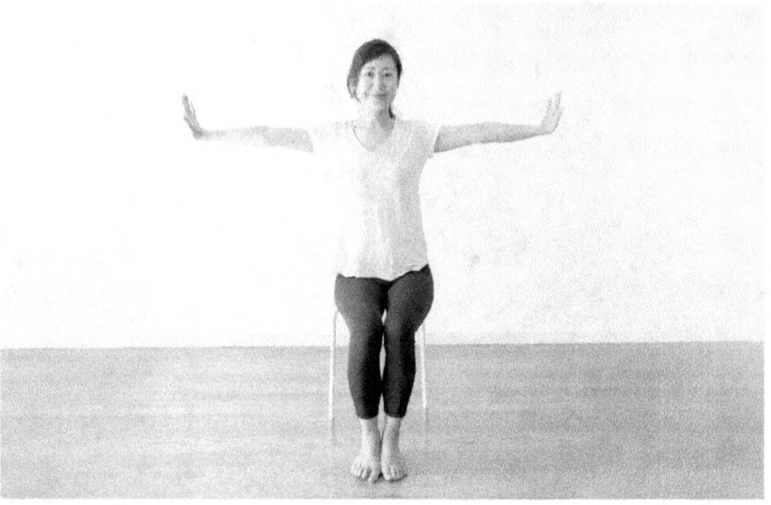

8.13: Virbhadrasana I

- Start in Seated Mountain and inhale deeply. Lift your upper body to the outside as you inhale, then bring your hands together over your head.

- As you aim straight up at the ceiling, lace your index and middle fingers together while keeping your thumbs and pointer fingers out.

- Roll your arms away from your ears as you exhale, allowing your shoulder blades to descend your back. This will activate the shoulder capsule, which comprises the muscles that stabilize your shoulder joint.

- As you settle down, keep inhaling deeply and evenly. Take at least five deep breaths before releasing your joined hands and letting your arms slowly fall back to your sides.

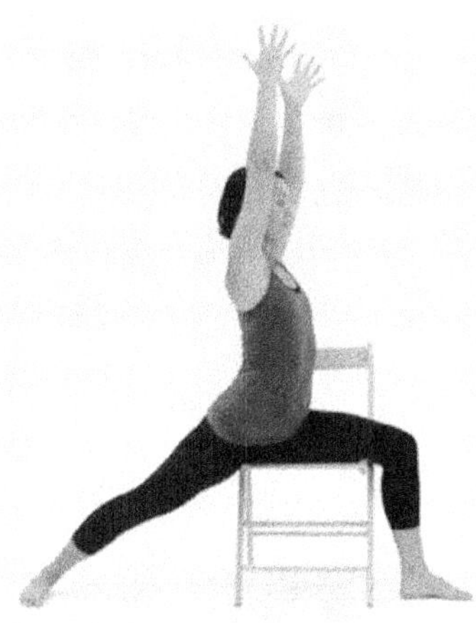

8.14: Paschimottanasana

- Fold your legs over after taking a deep breath in Seated Mountain while concentrating on lengthening your spine. For a little more support, you may start your hands on the bottoms of your feet and slide them along onto the floor as you fold, or you can maintain your hands at the sides as you go toward placing your body on your thighs.

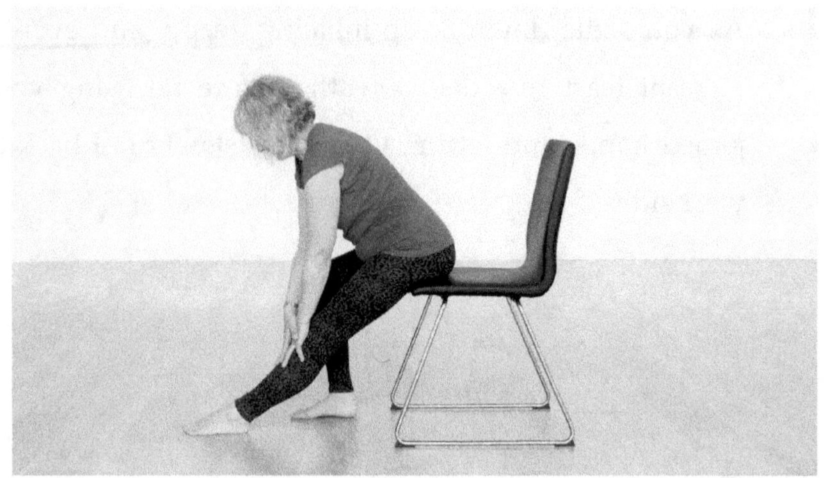

- In this position, take five or more slow, even breaths. It also passively lengthens your spine and stretches your back muscles while massaging your intestines to aid digestion.

- When you're ready, take a deep breath and raise your torso.

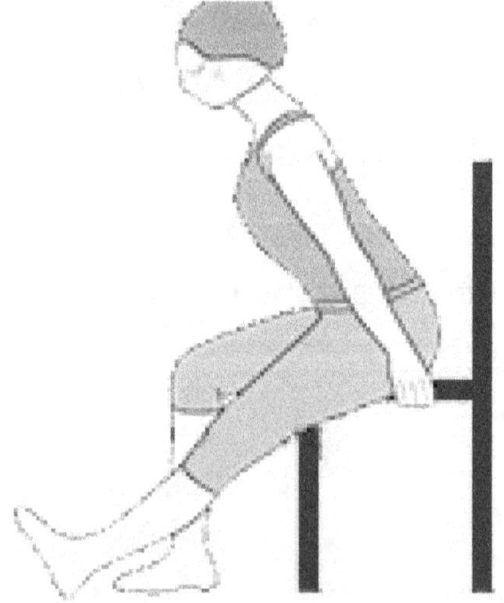

8.15: Garudasana Arms

As your shoulder joint is stabilized and flexed in this position, your arms and upper back are relaxed.

- As you inhale, extend your forearms out to the sides. Take a breath.

- Swing your right arm beneath your left and grip your shoulders using the opposite hands as you exhale to hug yourself.

- If your shoulders are more flexible, you may let go of your grasp and keep encircling your forearms until your right fingers rest in your left palm.

- Lift the elbows a couple of inches higher while inhaling.

- Rolling your shoulders away from the ears while exhaling will relax them.

- Take a few deep breaths and, if you'd like, repeat the shoulder roll and elbow raise.

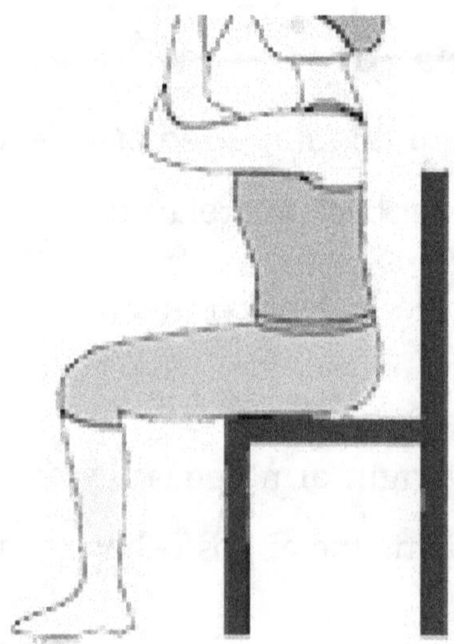

8.16: Backward Arm Hold

This may assist with posture, tension, and breathing issues by stretching your shoulders and opening your chest.

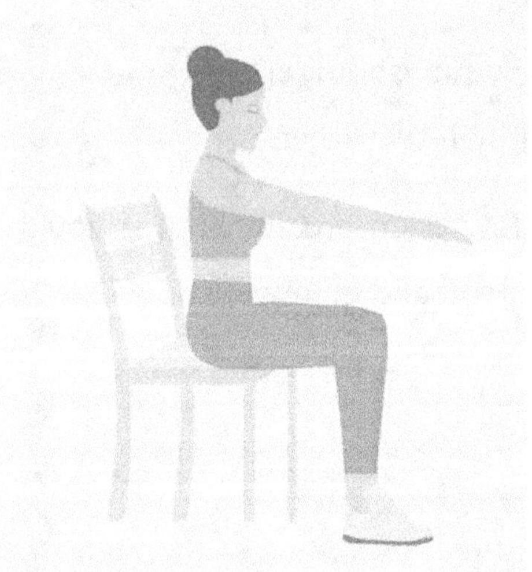

- Palms facing down, extend both arms toward the sides as you breathe.

- When you exhale, rotate your shoulders slightly forward so your palms face backward. Next, bend your forearms and let them swing across your back.

- You may keep your hands together using your fingertips, wrists, or elbows. Gently move your hands apart while maintaining your grip.

- Take note of which side it is if you hold onto your wrist or elbow.

- This time, grasp one wrist or elbow again and hold for five calm and even breaths.

- Then, release the clasp and repeat the exercise with the other arm.

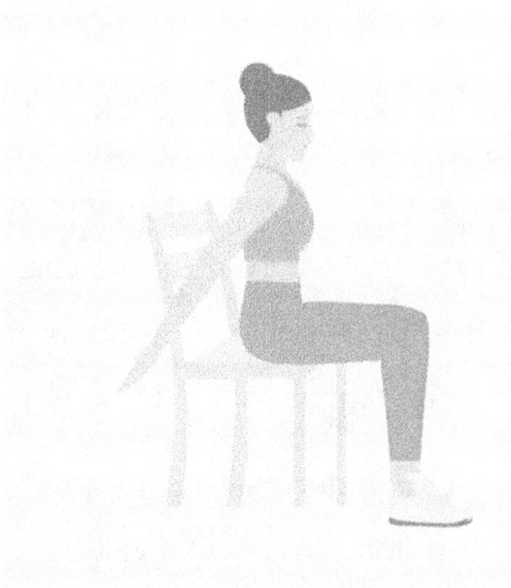

8.17: Simple Seated Twist

Twisting positions promote healthy circulation and digestion while easing lower back discomfort. They are often known as "detox" positions.

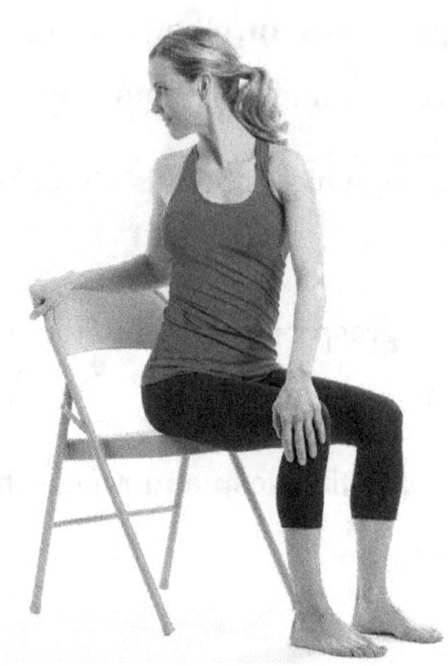

- Extend your spine once more as you inhale.

- With your arms at your sides and your right hand resting on the highest point of the chair's back, slowly rotate your upper torso to the right as you exhale. Your left arm will remain at your side.

- Take a right-shoulder glance. Hold onto the chair with your hands to maintain your twist but avoid making it deeper.

- Loosen this twist and face the front after five breaths. Continue on your left arm.

8.18: Janu Sirsasana

For this one, you can go closer to the tip of your seat. Just make sure you're seated firmly enough to prevent falling off.

- Sit straight with your right leg extended and your heel resting on the floor with your toes facing up. The closer you are to the front of the seat, the higher your portion may be. But once again, consider your support before bending forward.

- Place your hands on your extended leg. While exhaling, bend over the opposite leg while sliding your palms down the leg. As you inhale, lift through your spine.

- You may extend the stretch as much as you'd like if you're not pushing or straining and still feel supported by your seat and your hands. Consider grabbing the back portion of your leg or ankle to see if you can extend your reach further on your leg.

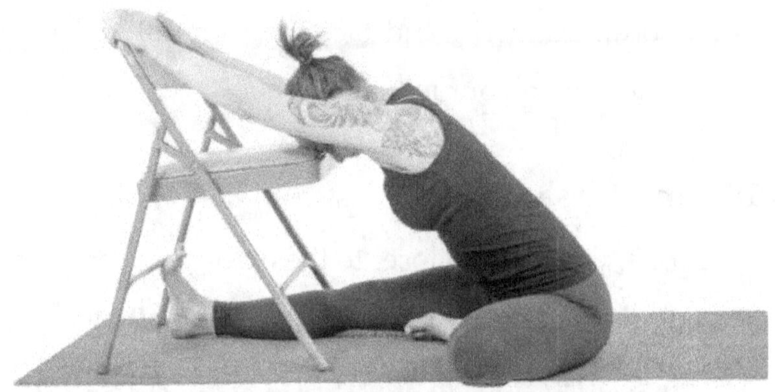

- Release the posture by employing an inhalation to assist you in rising after inhaling slowly and evenly five times, gradually descending each time. Repeat this position without your left leg extended, ensuring your torso is securely seated on the leading edge of the seat and realigning the knee of your right leg over the ankle before bending over. You can also do the same exercise with a pillow.

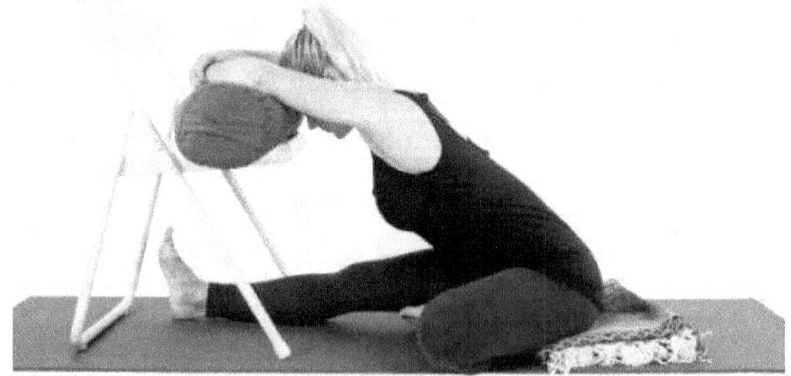

Chapter 9: Breathing Exercises

Breath is another of our most effective instruments for altering our mental state. Have you ever observed that you hold your breath when you're anxious or upset? Or perhaps you breathe quickly and shallowly because you're always rushing. Practicing how to inhale properly can have a significant positive impact on our physical condition and overall well-being, in addition to our mental health. Exercise is simpler as well with the proper psychological and physical preparation. We do breathe drills for chair yoga because of this.

9.1: Lips-Purse Breathing

This easy breathing technique enables you to slow back your breathing pace. You can practice breathing with a pursed lip at any moment. It might be especially helpful when bending, lifting, or climbing stairs. To properly learn the breathing pattern, practice taking this breath 4 to 5 times daily when you first start.

To do it:

1. Relax your neck, your shoulders.

2. Inhale slowly for two counts via your nose while keeping your mouth shut.

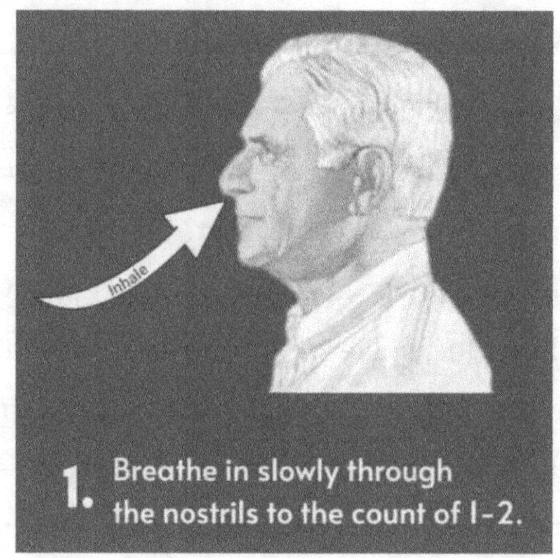

3. Lips should be puckered or pursed as if you were about to whistle.

4. Slowly exhale by blowing air between your pursed lips for a count of four.

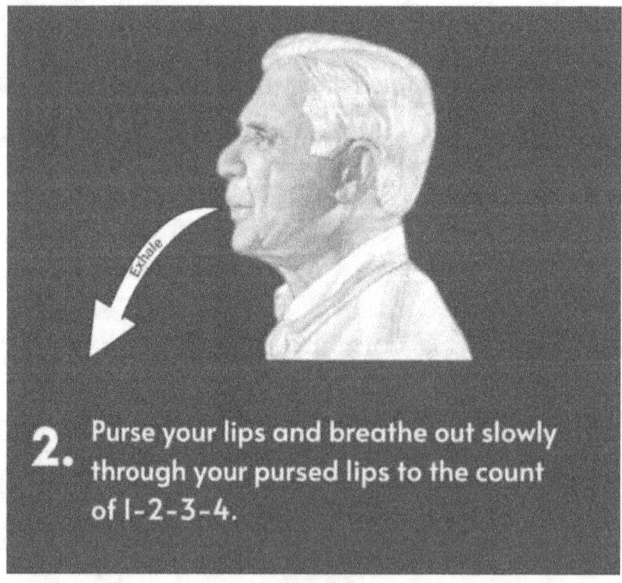

9.2: Diaphragmatic Breathing

Diaphragmatic breathing might help people use their diaphragm appropriately. A meta-analysis from 2020According to Trusted Source, this breathing method is especially beneficial for people who have trouble breathing because of cancer, heart issues, or chronic obstructive respiratory disease (COPD). It may also assist in relieving stress and help with eating disorders, diarrhea, elevated cholesterol levels, migraine attacks, and other medical conditions. Engage in 5–10 minutes of diaphragmatic breathing three–four times per day. You can feel exhausted when you start, but the method should get easier and seem more natural with practice.

To do this:

1. Place a pillow under your head and lie on your side with your knee slightly bent.

2. For support, you can put a pillow below your knees.

3. You may feel the mobility of your diaphragm by placing one palm on your lower chest and the other below your ribs.

4. Feel your stomach pushing into your hand.

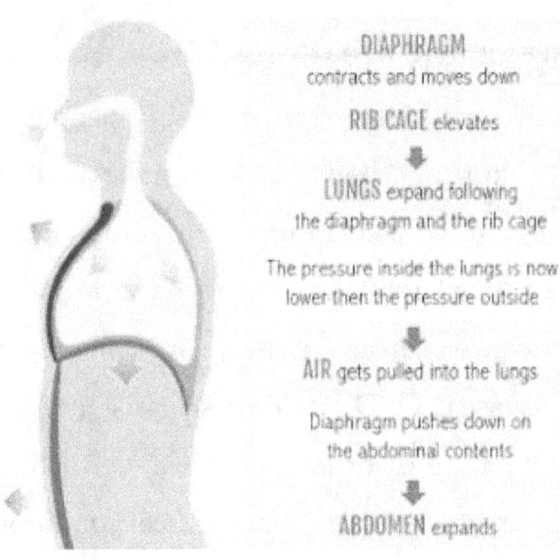

5. Try to keep the other hand still as much as you can.

6. Purse your lips as you exhale and contract your abdominals, keeping your top hand still.

7. One can place a paperback on your belly to make the activity more difficult. Once you've mastered belly breathing while lying lower, you can make it more challenging by attempting it while seated. After that, you can put the technique into practice while going about your daily business.

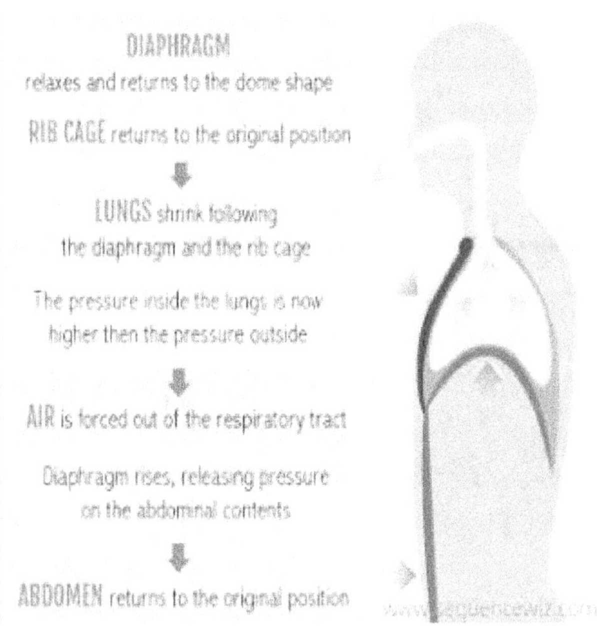

9.3: The Breath-Focus Method

This method of deep breathing uses focus words & phrases or imagery. You can pick a focus keyword that cheers you up, makes you feel at ease, or is neutral. Possibilities include harmony, letting go and relaxation, but they can be any term that allows you to concentrate on and repeat. As we build up your breathing focus action, you can commence with a 10-minute practice. Gradually extend the frequency until your treatments are at least 15-20 minutes.

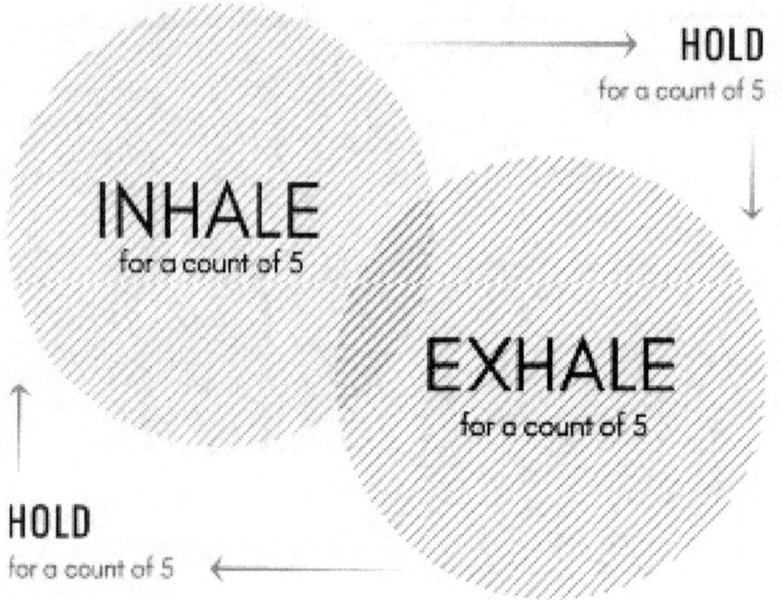

To perform:

1. Sit and lie up in a pleasant place.

2. Without attempting to alter your breathing, bring your attention to your breaths.

3. Several times, switch between taking regular breaths and deep ones. Notice any differences between normal breathing and lengthy breathing. Notice how the torso expands with strong inhalations.

4. Note how rapid breathing feels when compared to prolonged inhalation.

5. Practice your deep inhaling for a few moments.

6. Insert one hand beneath your abdomen button, keeping my belly comfortable, and notice how it elevates with each breath and falls with every exhale.

7. Let off a loud moan with every exhale.

8. Begin breathing focus by pairing this deep respiration with visuals and a focal word or sentence that will aid relaxation.

9.4: Lion's Breath

Lion's Breathe is an energetic yoga breathing meditation that is claimed to relieve tightness in your breast and face. It's also recognized in yoga called Lion's Pose.

To do this:

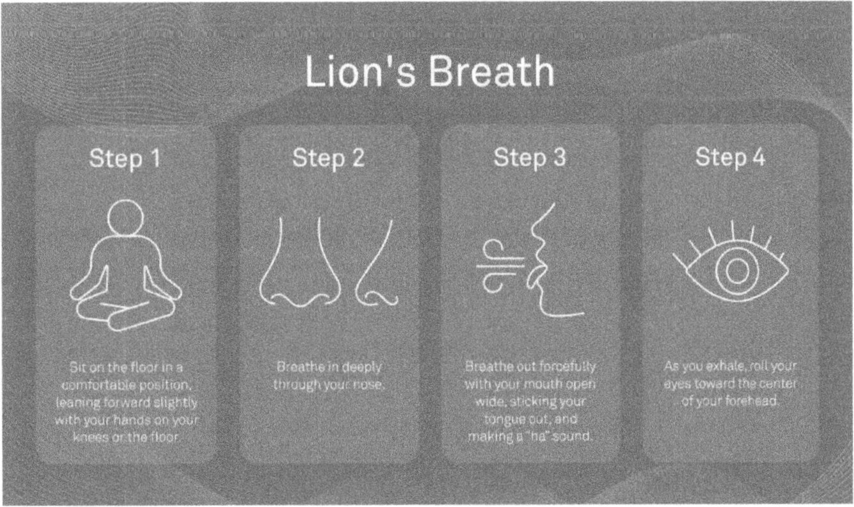

1. Move into a comfortable seating position. You can sit up
    on your feet or cross your legs.

2. Press your palms towards your knees, and your fingers
    extended wide.

3. Inhale deeply with your nose while widening your eyes
    wide.

4. At the identical time, open your jaw wide and stick out
    the end of your tongue, dragging the tip down towards
    your chin.

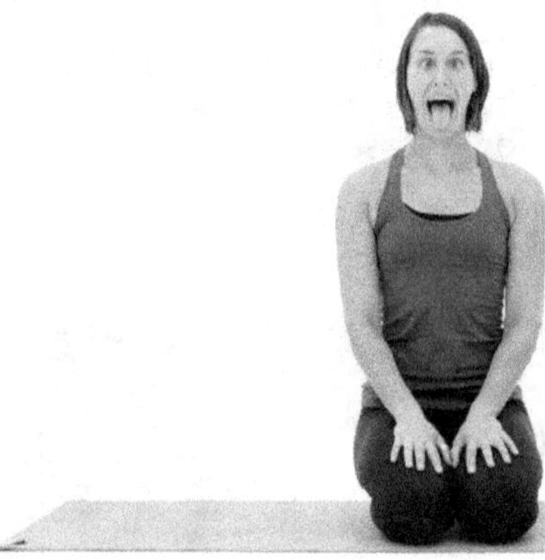

5. Compress the muscle groups at the top of your chest as
    you breathe through your mouth with a long "haaa"
    noise.

6. You can turn your head to look at the region behind your
    eyebrows or toward the tip of your nostril.

7. Do this inhalation 2 to 3 more.

9.5: Alternative Nostril Breathing

Alternative nostril blowing to boost cardiovascular function and decrease the heart rate. Nadi Shodhana is most effective on a stomach full. Avoid this routine if you've become sick or congested. Keep your breath soft and even through the practice.

To do this:

1. Adopt a comfortable sitting position.

2. Lift your right arm toward the bridge of your mouth, pressing your primary and middle fingers into your palm and letting the remaining fingers extend.

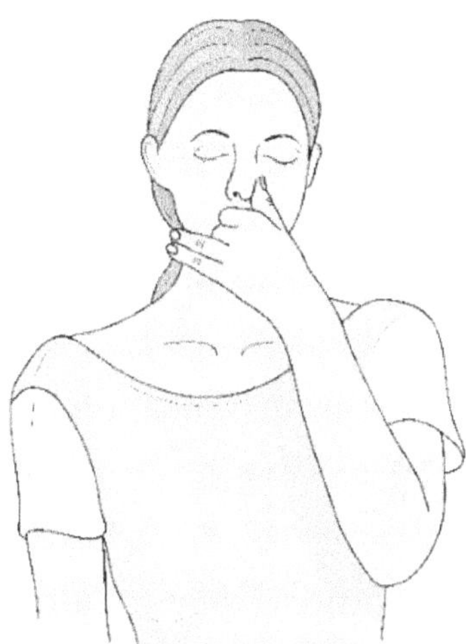

3. After letting out a breath, use your right hand to gently shut your right nostril.

4. Breathe into your left nostril and subsequently cover your left nostril between your opposite pinky or ring fingers.

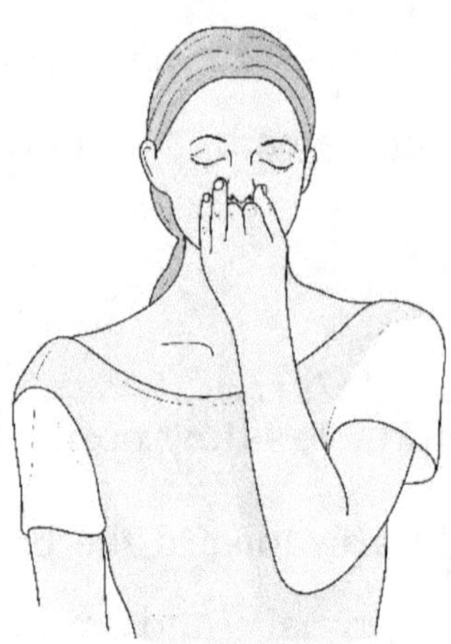

5. Lift your thumb and breath out through the opposite nostril.

6. Inhale into the right nostril and afterward close this nostril.

7. Release your hands to expose your left nostril & exhale via this side.

8. That is one cycle.

9. For up to five minutes, keep inhaling in this manner.

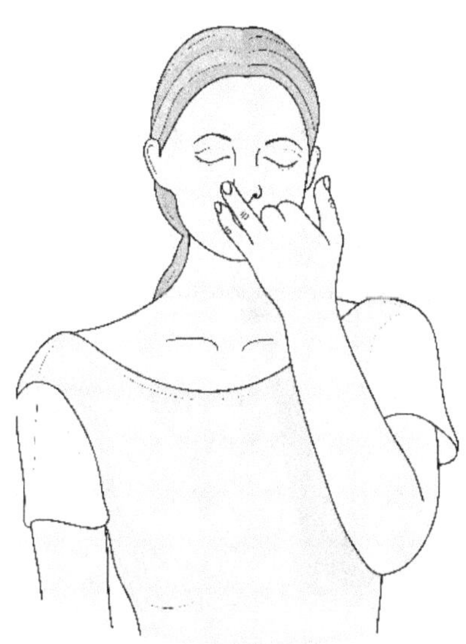

10. Finish your workout with an exhalation on the left hand.

9.6: Equal Breathing

Equal inhalation has been referred to as Sama Vritti in Sanskrit. This breathing exercise aims to equalize the length of your inhales and exhales. Making the air you breathe smooth and steady might assist in bringing about balance or composure. Research on older persons with high cholesterol levels found that this approach may assist in promoting mental well-being the increase the flow of oxygen to their minds and lungs.

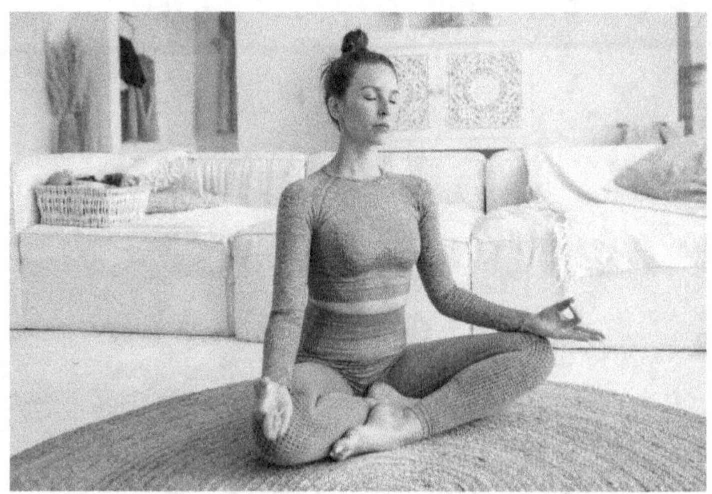

Select an inhalation length that is right—not too easy or hard. To keep it throughout the session, you also don't want it to be moving too quickly. Usually, this is from 3 and 5 counts. Once you get acclimated to equal breathing once seated, you can perform it during your daily yoga routine or other daily tasks.

To perform:

1. Adopt a chair.

2. Inhale in and out from your nose.

3. Count throughout each breath and exhale to be sure they are even in time. On the other hand, choose a single letter or brief phrase to repeat with each inhalation and exhale.

4. If it makes you more comfortable, you might include a small pause for breath storage after each inhalation and exhalation.

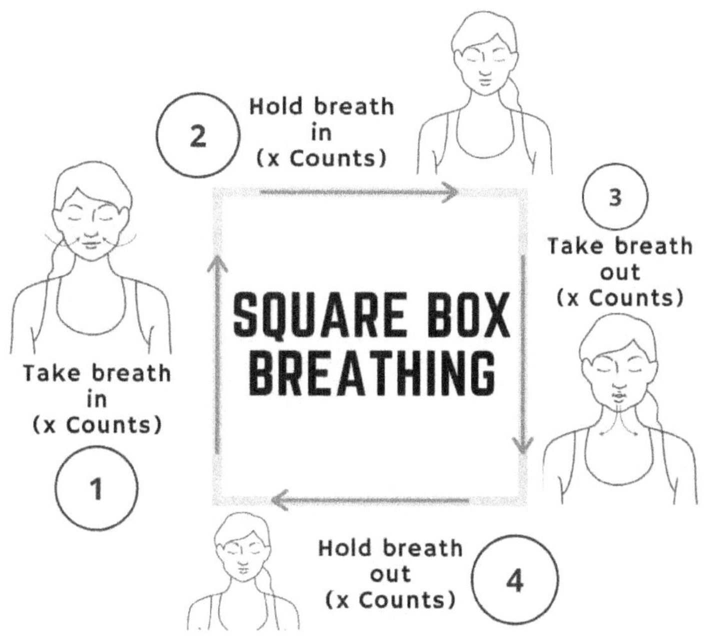

9.7: Resonant Breathing

When you inhale at a rate of 5 complete breaths per minute, you engage in resonant breathing, also called coherent breathing. This rate can be attained by counting five on the inhale and the exhale of each breath. This rate of breathing increases your cardiovascular variability (HRV), lowers your stress levels, and, according to a study published in 2017, can alleviate the symptoms of depressive disorder when utilized alongside Iyengar yoga.

To accomplish this:

1. Take a deep breath for the count of 5, then let it out simultaneously.

2. Maintain this breathing rhythm for at least a few minutes at a minimum.

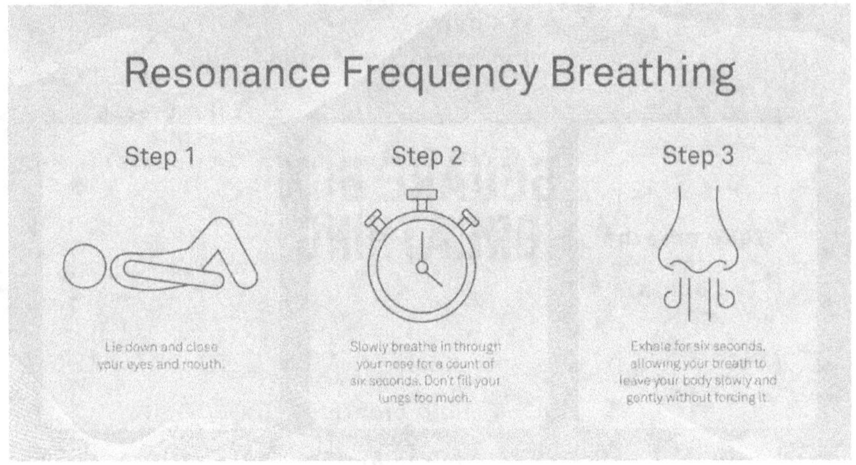

9.8: Sitali Breath

This yoga breathing technique helps you calm your internal temperature and simultaneously calm your mind and body. You should try to slightly lengthen the duration of your breath without forcing it. Because Sitali breath requires you to inhale through your mouth, you should probably practice in an environment that does not contain any allergies that you are sensitive to and does not have an elevated level of air pollution.

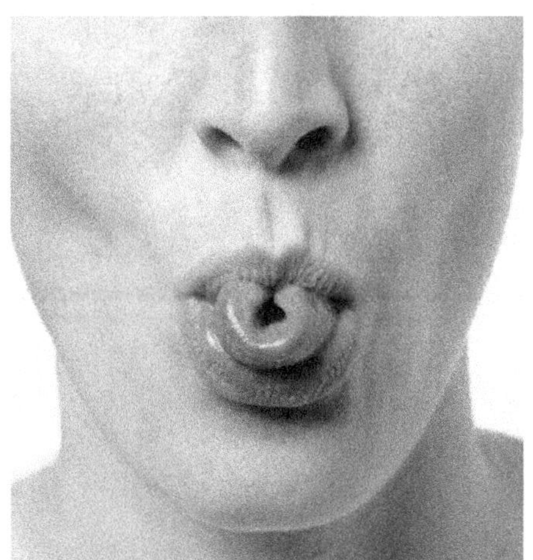

To accomplish this:

1. Find a position that allows you to sit comfortably.

2. Your tongue should be sticking out, and you should curl it to bring the outer edges together.

3. You might try pursing your lips instead if this doesn't work with your tongue.

4. Take a deep breath through your mouth.

5. Exhale completely through your nostrils when you do so.

6. You should keep inhaling in this manner for up to five minutes.

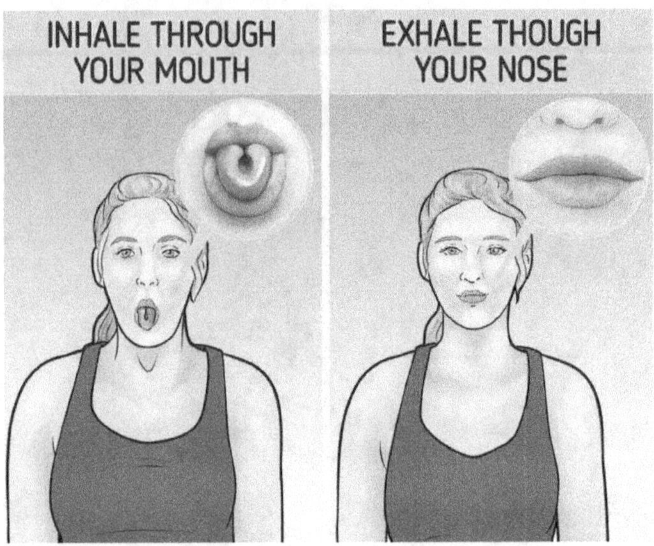

9.9: Deep Breathing

By releasing any air that may have become stuck in the pulmonary system and allowing you to take in more oxygen-rich air, deep breathing can help alleviate the symptoms of air loss. It is possible that doing so will assist you in feeling more relaxed and grounded.

To accomplish this:

1. Pull your elbows back and slightly to the side while sitting or standing to give your chest room to expand.

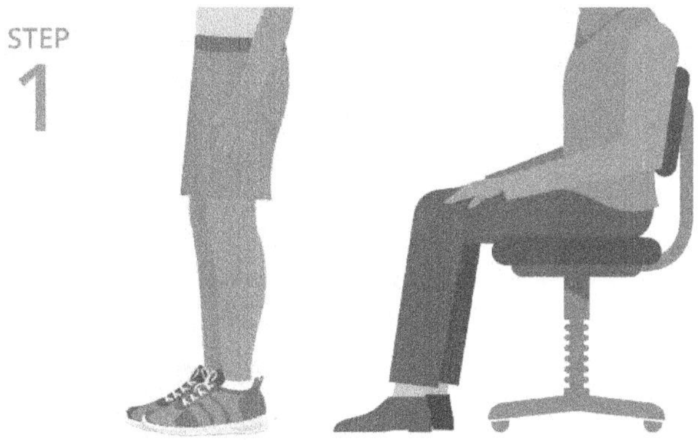

2. Inhale fully through your nose and let the air fill your lungs.

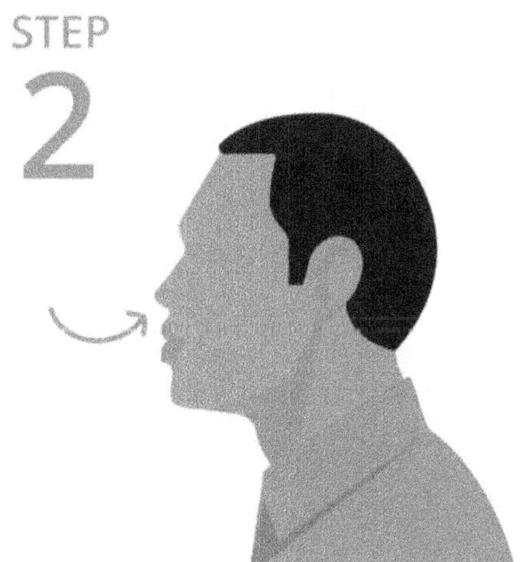

3. Hold your breath until the count of five has passed.

4. Exhale via your nose as you slowly let the air out of your body.

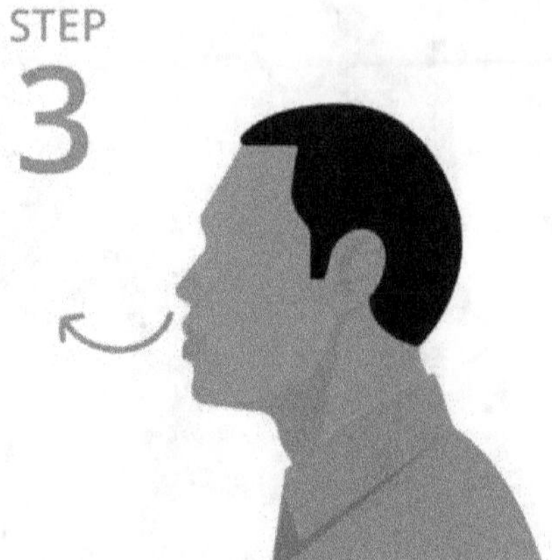

Hold your breath and count to
3 then exhale

The one-of-a-kind sensation from this yoga breathing exercise helps establish instant tranquility and is especially calming for the area around your forehead. Some people find it effective to relieve their annoyance, anxiety, or rage with humming bee breath. According to research, it may help slow your heart rate, improve your ability to think clearly and make you less angry or agitated. The best environment to practice this would be one in which you would not be interrupted if you were to hum.

To accomplish this:

1. Find a position that allows you to sit comfortably.

2. Put your eyes out and loosen the muscles in your face.

3. Put the first fingers of your firsthand on the tragus cartilage, which is the cartilage that partially conceals your ear canal.

4. After breathing in, exhale while softly pressing your fingertips into the cartilage.

5. Make a very loud buzzing sound while keeping your mouth closed.

6. Keep going for as long as you feel fine doing it.

Chapter 10: Chair Yoga Workout Plans

You may feel the life-altering effects of yoga in a noticeably brief time while remaining seated in the ease and convenience of your chair. This program is ideal for those with restricted mobility, people who work in offices, or anyone looking for a simple and accessible approach to include mindful movement and meditation in their everyday lives. This program consists of exercises focusing on different body parts to increase strength, flexibility, and a sensation of serenity. Therefore, locate a comfortable place to sit, focus on your core, and be ready to improve your health and well-being. You may create a healthier body, a more serene mind, and a more joyous spirit by devoting only ten minutes daily to this chair yoga practice. All you need to do is sit in the chair. Let's go on this life-changing trip together, shall we?

10.1: 10 Minute Plan

The following chair yoga program takes 10 minutes each day:

1. **Take two minutes to sit tall and breathe.**

- Sit in an armchair with your feet flat on the floor and your back straight.

- Shut your eyes and inhale through your nostrils and exhale through your mouth for a few deep breaths.

- With each breath, concentrate on lengthening your spine or relaxing your shoulders.

2. **Neck stretches (one minute)**

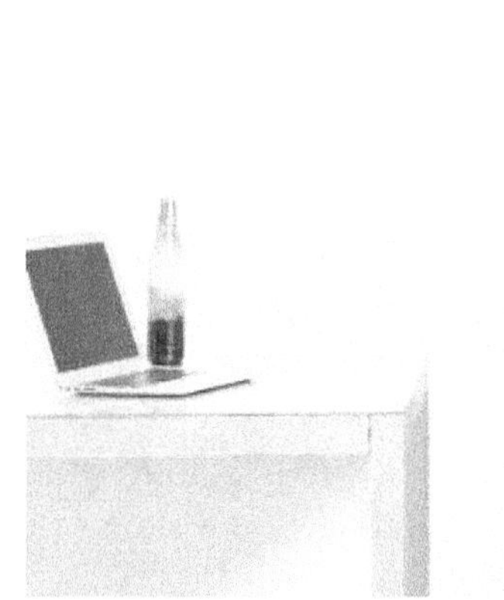 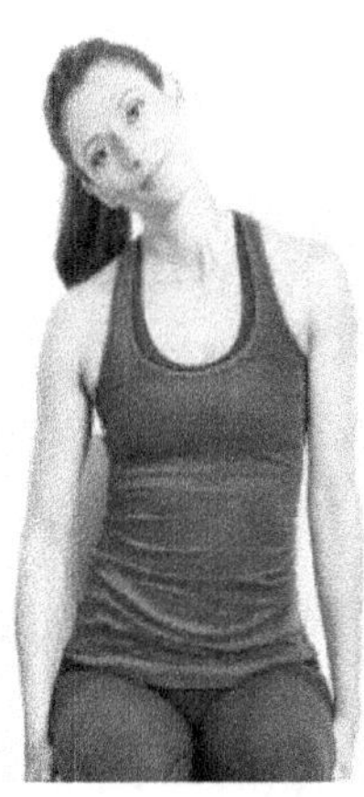

- Tilt your head slightly to the right, close your right ear to your right shoulder.

- Repeat for the left side after holding for a little while.

- Keep changing sides to further loosen the neck tissues and stretch them.

3. A two-minute seated cat-and-cow stretch

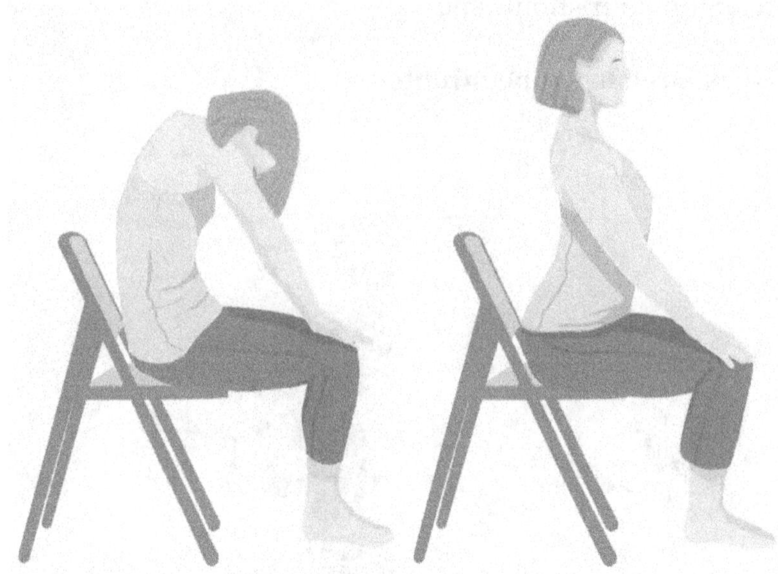

- Put both hands on your thighs or knees.

- Exhale as you elevate your chest, arch your spine, and do the cow stance.

- As you exhale, adopt the cat stance by arching your back and lowering your jaw to your chest.

- Using your breath, go between the cow and cat postures while letting your spine gradually flex.

4. Seated Forward Folding (2 minutes)

- Place your feet firmly on the ground while sitting at the front of the chair.

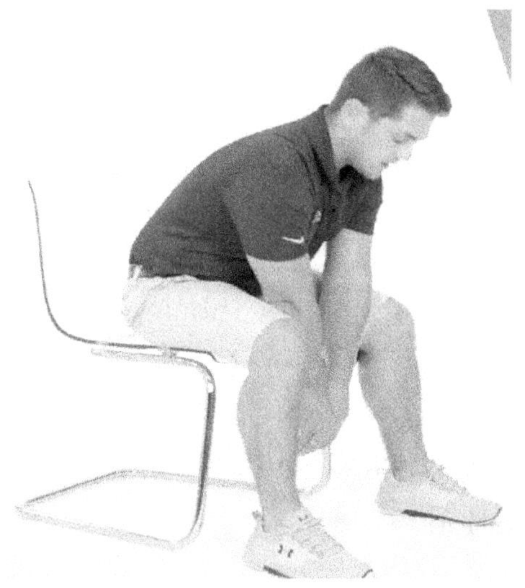

- Take a deep breath, stretch your spine, and raise your arms.

- Taking a deep breath out, bend forward from the hips and place your hands or fingers on the ground or your shins.

- Hold the forward fold while inhaling deeply and feeling your back or hamstrings gently stretch.

5. **Seated Bend (2 minutes)**

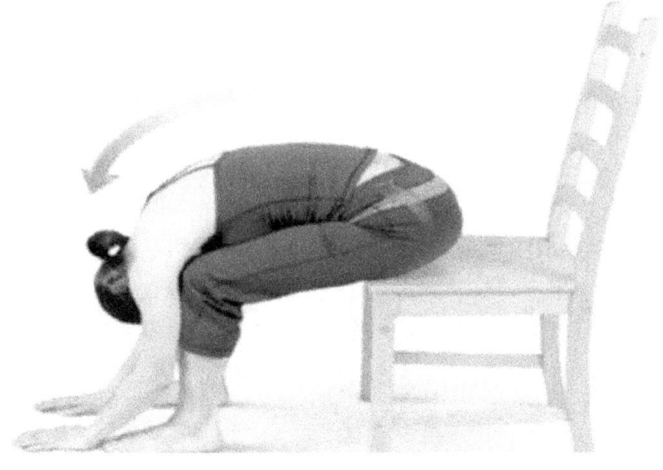

- Sit tall, place your hands on your thighs, and flat your toes on the floor.

- Exhale while twisting to the right, keeping your right hand firmly on the chair's back and your left hand around the exterior of your right foot. Inhale while lengthening your spine.

- Hold the twist while inhaling deeply and feeling the spine's gradual rotation.

- Repeat the rotation on the left side with your left hand resting on the chair's back and the other hand on the exterior of your left leg.

6. **Seated Head Rolls (1 minute)**

- Rotate your shoulders clockwise up, back, downward, and forward.

- Pay attention to relaxing any stiffness in your neck and shoulder region.

- Reverse the shoulder rolls' motion.

7. **Sitting Mindful Breathing (one minute)**

- Sit quietly with your torso straight and your eyes closed.

- Put your hands around your tummy and breathe through your nose slowly and deeply.

- Feel your tummy expand as you inhale and contract as you exhale.

- Pay attention to your breathing and eliminate any ideas or other distractions to be truly present.

8. **Complete for one minute in Savasana (Corpse Pose)**

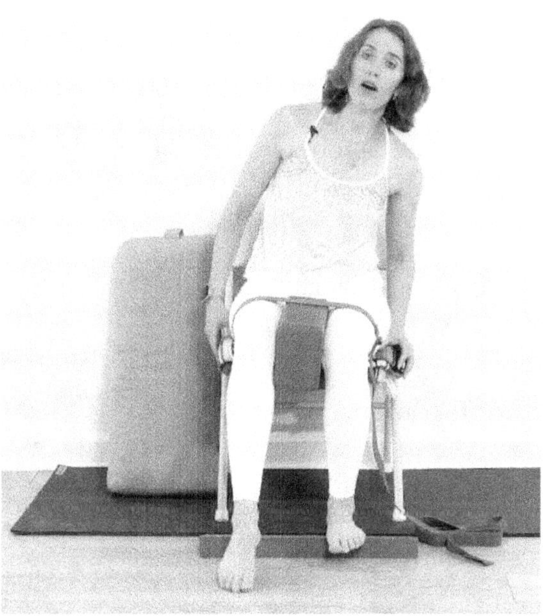

- Close your eyes and relax your eyes while sitting comfortably.

- Let go of all stress and give yourself up to total relaxation.

- Before continuing with the remainder of your day, use this time to relax and recharge.

Remember that you may modify this procedure to suit your requirements and tastes. You may practice additional postures or hold each stance longer if you have extra time. You may benefit from chair yoga's physical and psychological effects by regularly implementing this 10-minute daily program into your calendar.

10.2: One-Week Plan (With Alternative Exercises)

Sure! Here's a one-week chair yoga plan with 10 minutes of practice each day:

10.2.1: Day 1

Warm-up: Start with 1-minute-deep breathing using the Lips-Purse Breathing technique (9.1).

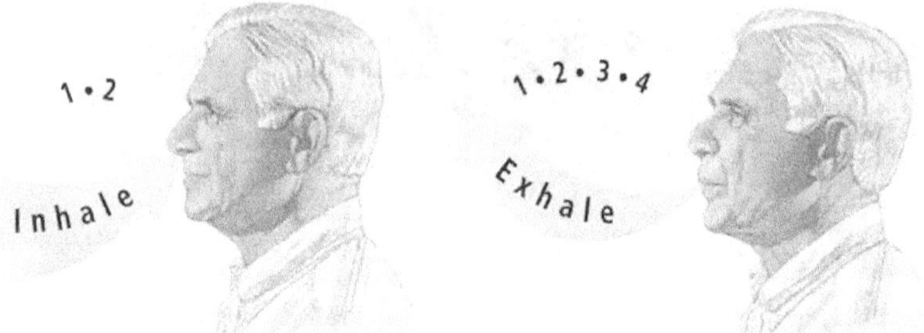

Pose: Cat-Cow Stretch - Spend 5 minutes alternating between the cow and cat poses, syncing the movements with your breath.

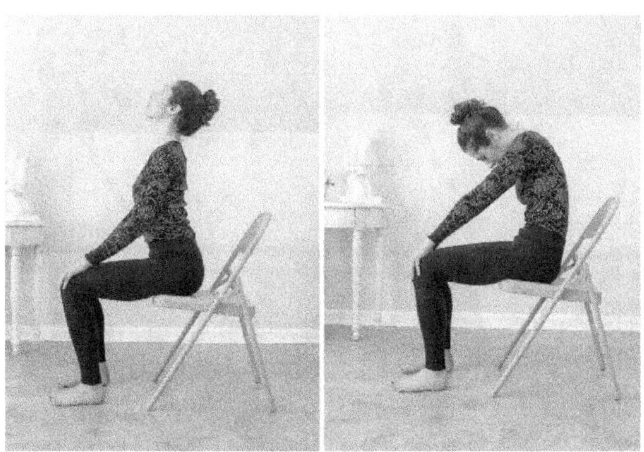

Cool-down: Finish with 1 minute of relaxation in Chair Savasana.

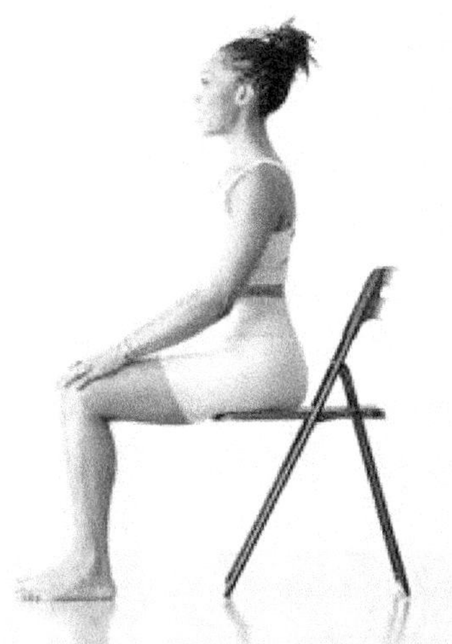

10.2.2: Day 2

Warm-up: 1 minute of deep breathing with Diaphragmatic Breathing.

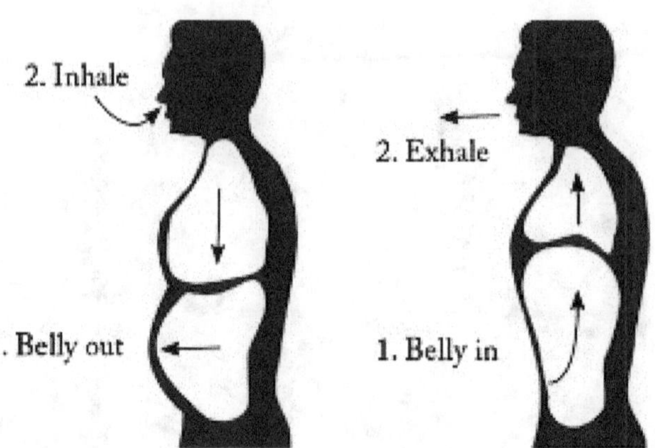

Pose: Urdhva Hastasana - Practice this poses for 5 minutes, focusing on maintaining good posture and extending your arms toward the ceiling.

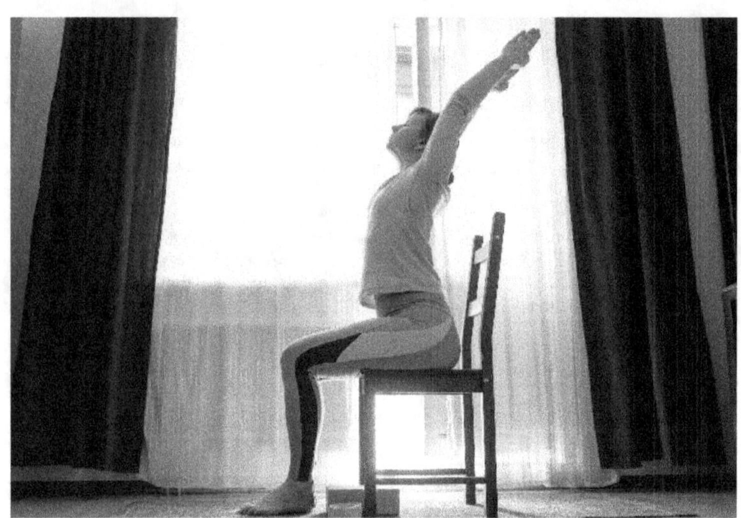

Cool-down: 1 minute of relaxation in Chair Savasana.

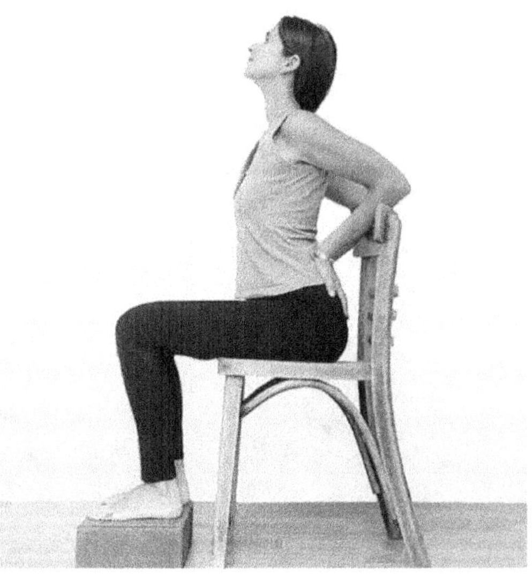

10.2.3: Day 3

Warm-up: 1 minute of deep breathing with the Breath-Focus Method.

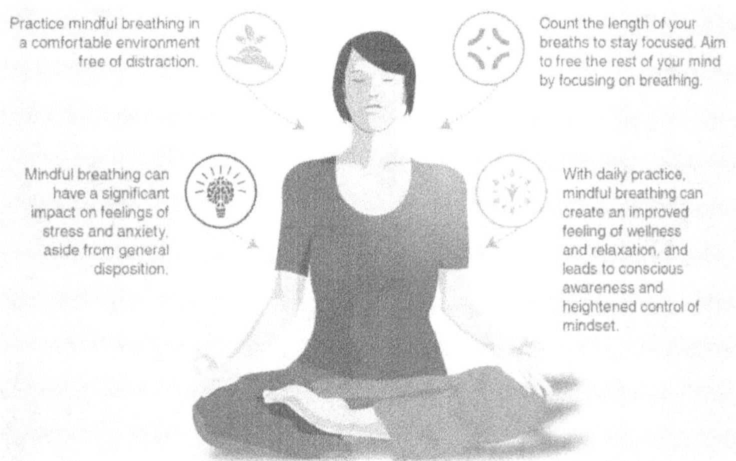

Pose: Chair Forward Bend - Spend 5 minutes practicing this pose, exhaling as you bend over your legs.

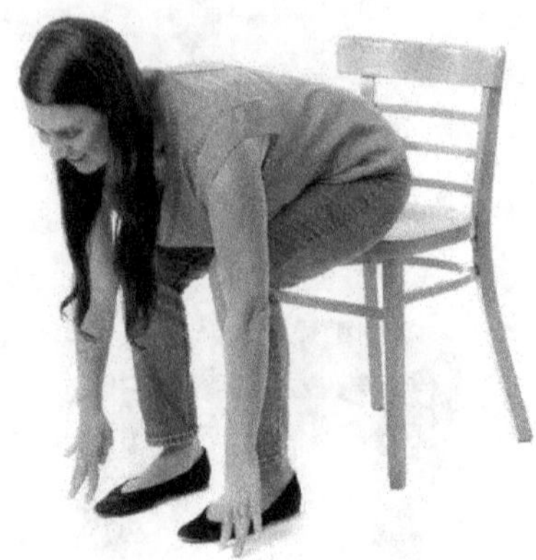

Cool-down: 1 minute of relaxation in Chair Savasana.

10.2.4: Day 4

Warm-up: 1 minute of deep breathing with Lion's Breath.

Pose: Extended Side Angle Pose - Practice this poses for 5 minutes on each side, focusing on the deep breaths and opening your chest.

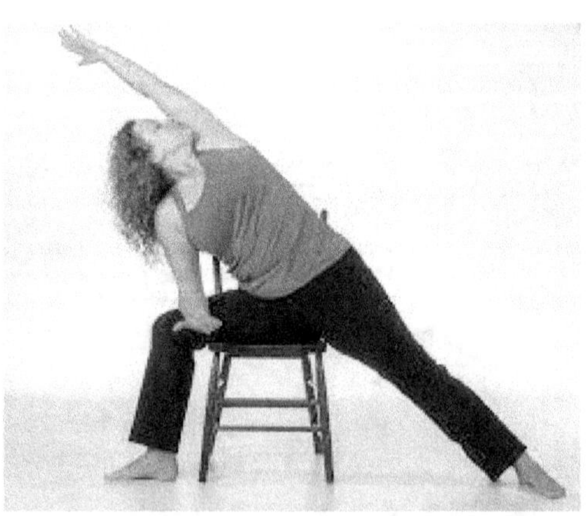

Cool-down: 1 minute of relaxation in Chair Savasana.

10.2.5: Day 5

Warm-up: 1 minute of deep breathing with Alternative Nostril Breathing.

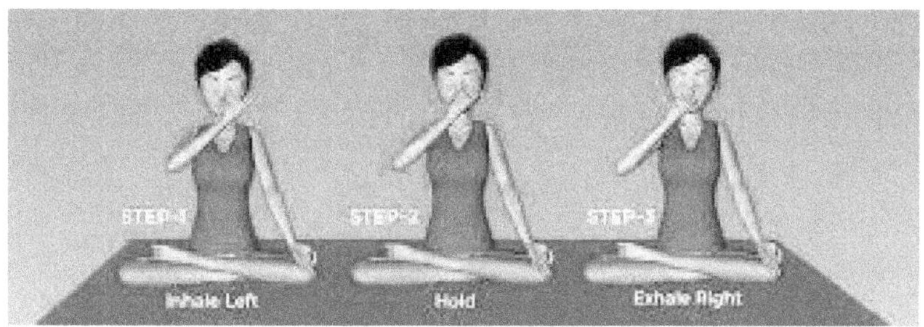

Pose: Chair Pigeon - Spend 5 minutes on each leg, maintaining the posture and exploring a gentle forward lean for a deeper stretch.

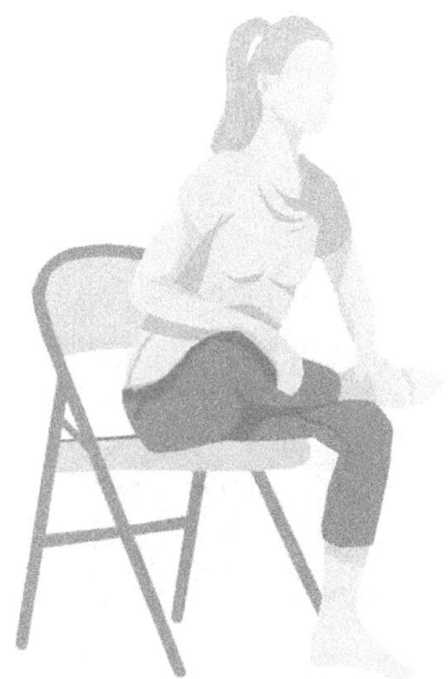

Cool-down: 1 minute of relaxation in Chair Savasana.

10.2.6: Day 6

Warm-up: 1 minute of deep breathing with Equal Breathing.

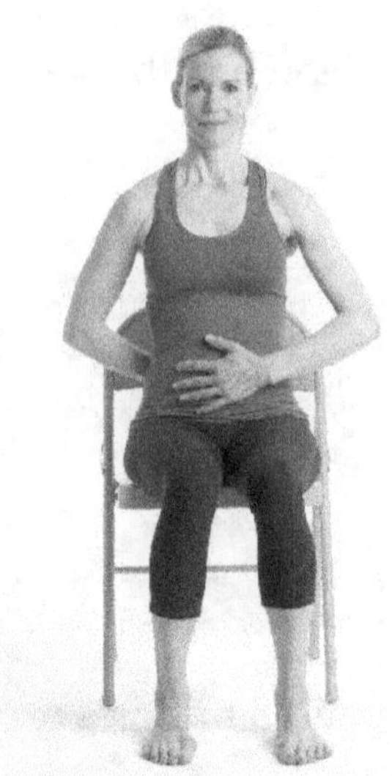

Pose: Chair Eagle - Practice this poses for 5 minutes, focusing on crossing your legs and arms and maintaining balance.

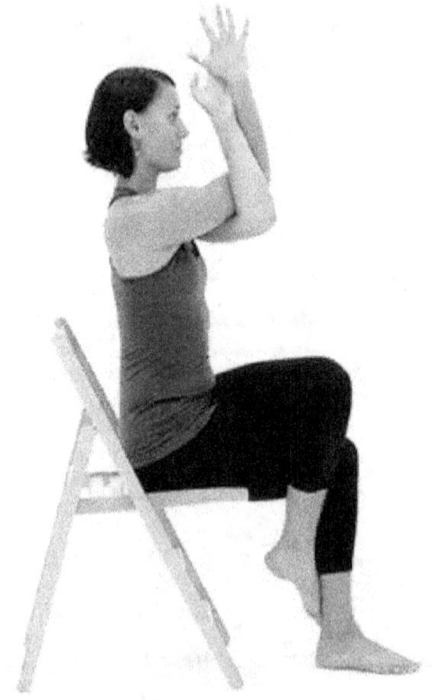

Cool-down: 1 minute of relaxation in Chair Savasana.

10.2.7: Day 7

Warm-up: 1 minute of deep breathing with Lips-Purse Breathing.

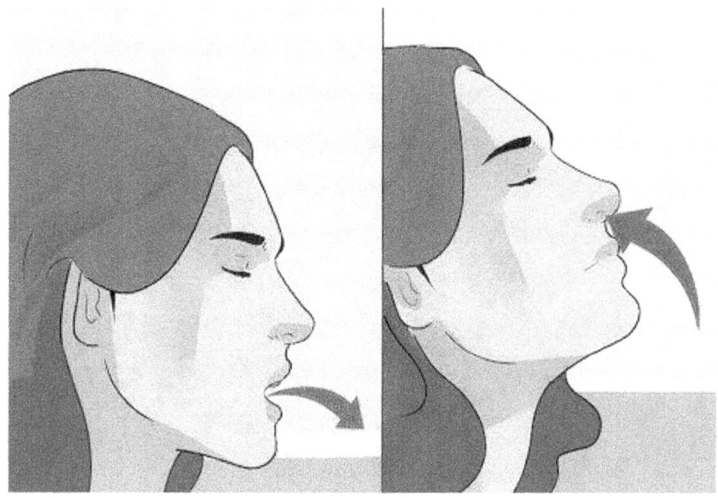

Pose: Chair Spinal Twist- Spend 5 minutes on each side, twisting your upper body and maintaining the pose.

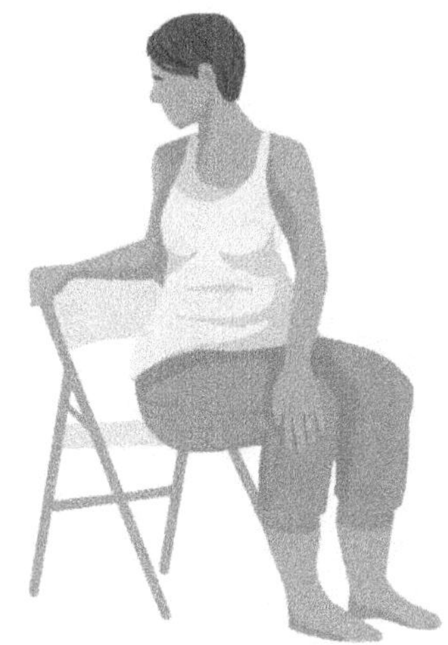

Cool-down: 1 minute of relaxation in Chair Savasana.

Remember to listen to your body, modify the poses as needed, and always prioritize your safety and comfort during the practice. Enjoy your week of chair yoga!

Conclusion

This book has examined using a chair to support mindfulness mobility yoga. It has offered a thorough warm-up program that aids in waking up and energizing the whole body. The book provides a secure and convenient alternative for people of any age or level of fitness to practice yoga by emphasizing deep breathing, moderate movements, and modifying conventional yoga positions to be done using a chair.

The described modified postures, including Chair Tree Pose, Armchair Warrior 3, Chairs Revolved Triangle, Suspended Half Moon, Armchair Pose, and Chair Lunge, among others, provide several advantages, including building the body, enhancing flexibility and balance, and encouraging relaxation and awareness. Each pose's step-by-step instructions guarantee appropriate alignment and make it simple for readers to do the exercises.

This book improves physical well-being and supports emotional and mental wellness by including mindful breathing and creating a feeling of presence. People may connect to their breath, let go of stress, and discover brief moments of peace and tranquility among the bustle of everyday life by engaging in mindful mobility yoga while sitting in a chair.

The book also stresses listening to your body and adapting as necessary, enabling people to customize their workouts to their capabilities and limits. It promotes a holistic strategy for health and well-being by fostering self-care and self-compassion.

The mindful movement yoga poses described in this book provide a gentle and efficient approach to nourishing the body, relaxing the mind, and fostering a feeling of well-being, whether done as a stand-alone program or as an introduction to other types of exercise. By adopting these practices into their everyday lives, readers may experience the transforming power of yoga even without a conventional mat or studio space.

In conclusion, utilizing a chair as a supporting tool, this book is an invaluable resource for anybody looking to integrate yoga and mindful movement into their life. It offers a basis for mindful mobility yoga that may improve mental, emotional, and physical health. Readers may start on an adventure of self-discovery, taking care of oneself and holistic development via yoga practice with the direction and adjustments offered.

Bonus

I am confident that using this information will enable you to improve your overall health and physical well-being. I sincerely thank you for purchasing my book. For more stimulation and a broader overview. I have included video courses, not mine, taken on you tube that I think are very valuable.

To access just click on the link for the eBook edition or scan the QR code on the next page.

Remember that perseverance pays off. Use the ten minutes of "exercise" every day.

With gratitude!

https://docs.google.com/document/d/1JiJH6_WMazi0pMF
pgRW6q1qJ10hHxZ50/edit